FIND YOUR WAY:
ILLNESS, DOCTORS,
AND HEALTHCARE

*A doctor's guide to
taking charge of your health and
navigating modern healthcare*

MARIA V GIBSON, MD, PHD

FERVENT PRESS

DISCLAIMER

This book details the author's personal opinions and experiences. All patient and doctors' names and identities have been changed to protect their privacy. This book is not intended to diagnose, treat, cure, or prevent any condition or disease. It is not intended as a substitute for consultation with a licensed healthcare practitioner. Consult with your own physician regarding opinions and suggestions made in this book before you begin any healthcare program, or change your lifestyle in any way. The author and publisher do not represent or warrant that the information accessible via this book is accurate, complete, or current.

Neither the author nor the publisher will be liable for damages of any kind relating to the use of this book. This book provides content related to physical and mental health issues. As such, the use of this book implies your acceptance of this disclaimer.

Enquiries: mariagibsonmd@gmail.com

Editorial: Claire McGregor, Jess Lomas
Cover and Interior Design: KUHN Design Group | kuhndesigngroup.com

ISBN 979-8-9876515-1-3 (paperback)
ISBN 979-8-9876515-0-6 (ebook)

To my children Vladimir and Anastasia,
who made life worth living

To my patients, who taught me to be a doctor

To my students and residents, who taught me to be a teacher

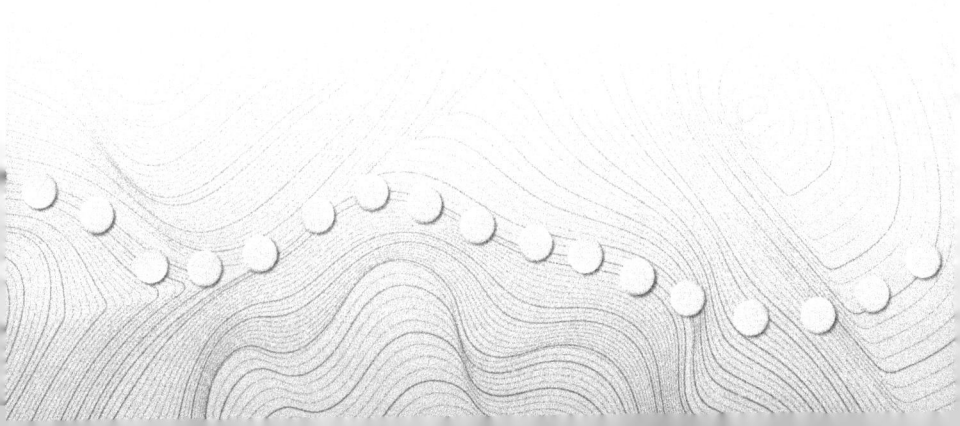

CONTENTS

PREFACE

After thirty-five years of listening to patients' experiences with illnesses and healthcare, and their relentless search for good doctors, practices and hospitals to restore their health, I realized the problem is not just about the resources or lack of available services, doctors or technology. Even those who are financially secure, with good health insurance, have difficulties maintaining their health and establishing mutually satisfying relationships in healthcare. You might think that in our society, where medical practices and doctors are available in every neighborhood, shopping center and online, we would not have a problem receiving sound medical advice and high-quality healthcare. Yet patients transfer their care from one practice to another, pay for concierge practices, opt for new models of "value-based care" in search of the "right" doctor who understands their struggles and their pursuits and who can safely guide them through their health journey.

Medicine and healthcare stopped being paternalistic long ago, where we relied on the ultimate trust of a physician's opinions, when patients unwearyingly accepted and followed their doctor's advice, without contemplation. Now, equipped with unlimited sources of information available online, we have been transformed from quiet "sufferers" to people who question doctors' opinions and look for faster, easier, cheaper, and more convenient and sustainable solutions to our health problems.

The time has passed when the patient-doctor relationship and trust determined the rules. Medicine has become technologically advanced, as well as a complicated and profitable business, with rules to protect the interests of many beyond patients and doctors. Many of us feel influenced by faceless bureaucracies, with their regulations that come above the purpose of patients seeking medical care and doctors who have dedicated their craft to provide it. The patient-doctor relationship has extended to the relationships within circles, which involves insurance companies, pharmacies, medical practice teams and administrators at different levels of the hierarchy within healthcare systems. Patients and doctors have to develop working relationships not only between each other—a challenge in itself—but also with these healthcare teams, to transform the doctors' advice into the reality of diagnosis and treatment.

This transformation in modern healthcare has required new skills from patients and their doctors to overcome the challenges these changes present, far from the previously simple patient and doctor interactions. Overwhelmed with discovered genetic loads, self-destructive behaviors, illnesses and longevity pursuits, patients try to get through the current barriers to the sources of wisdom, skills and experience of compassionate physicians to receive scientifically advanced medical care that is not only safe but also convenient. They have learned to study their healthcare records, search for medical information and "shop" for doctors, hospitals and treatments.

Doctors have been transformed into "providers," who, in addition to the lifelong learning of medicine, have to develop skills in electronic communication, telemedicine, and patient satisfaction, and speak a language of billing, coding, value-based quality metrics, and customer service.

There are no instructions on how to care about your health. Are my symptoms dangerous? Who should I tell about my symptoms and when? What online health information is reliable? Should I try dietary supplements before going to the doctor? Should I talk about all my problems when I've just met my new doctor?

There are also no instructions on how to navigate through changing healthcare. Medicine is a regulated and litigated business by the nature of the risks involved. Time has become a virtue that both patients and doctors must obey. During brief conversations, doctors need patients' help to come up with the correct diagnosis and treatment. Without this help, cues to diagnoses can be missed. Are patients ready to provide a meaningful medical history, which will point doctors to the right diagnosis? To substitute this informational gap, doctors may order more and more tests to bring clarity or offer more medications. This cascade of "overtreatment" could be prevented by patients providing a detailed, organized history and making shared decisions based on doctors' knowledge of science and patients' awareness of their bodies, habits and experiences. We all, doctors and patients alike, make mistakes. I learned as a doctor and a patient that medical mistakes will happen less if we watch out for our own medical care. But how do we do that?

There is no training for patients on how to be in charge of their health, when and where to seek medical advice or how to become doctors' partners. We learn this as we go through our or our loved one's struggles with illnesses and experiences with doctors and healthcare.

In this book, I have collected suggestions and recommendations that I wish my patients knew while looking for answers to medical questions, communicating with their doctors and medical teams, and making decisions about their health. This book is a guide on how to take charge of your health and build partnerships with your clinicians, so that decisions being made fit into your goals, culture, and budget. Through examples of my patients, who have taught me wisdom about patient-doctor communication, I will show you how to recognize and overcome the obstacles for your medical care by identifying your health footprints—your roots and medical history—and developing self-awareness about your risks, powers, and self-destructive behaviors. Through learning about your "normalcy" pattern, you will be able to recognize symptoms and signs of illness and spot the red flags that should prompt you to seek help. I will show you how to communicate your medical history in a form that both you and your doctor can understand, share, and use to make your visits efficient and productive.

This book will help you to find your way through illness and healthcare; when, how and where to seek answers to your medical questions, find the "right" doctor and how to navigate through medical offices and hospitals. In other words, I will show you how to create your healthcare map and use medical services to your advantage. When you know your way, you can take charge of your healthcare. You might think, "It's easier for a doctor to take charge of my health." But after three decades of doctoring, it was only after I stepped into my patients' shoes and felt the vulnerability of being sick, and the pressure of uncertainty or whether I would ever be cured, did I realize that we are the *owners of our bodies* and we *are in charge of our health*. We just have to find the way.

INTRODUCTION

"Turn your wounds into wisdom."

OPRAH WINFREY

Jazz music was playing quietly. Men and women in blue gowns were moving with the music, while connecting my body to the blinking monitors, asking if I was comfortable. There was a certain mystery about this room. The blinking monitors, large screens and imaging equipment of the cardiac catheterization lab kept secrets of many hearts. Reaching someone's heart by inserting a tiny tube into the blood vessel of an arm or leg and seeing the heart pushing the injected contrast material through the chambers, vessels, valves, then out through the aorta, the biggest human vessel, with predictable frequency is one of the most powerful pictures.

My visits to the hospital's cardiac catheterization lab had always been about my patients and the verdict of the cardiologists. This time, it was different. The large surgical lamp was shining right into *my* chest. It was I who lay on the surgical table connected to the monitors. My life rolled before me like a fast-forwarding movie: my children smiling and stretching their tiny hands toward me, and then all grown up, friends who seemed to never grow old, men I'd loved, and who seemed to magically continue to love me back, and patients I'd fought for against their army of illnesses.

I had a good run, I told myself, thinking about my life. *Quite an adventure*—referring mostly to 16 June 1996, when I pulled out my Russian roots to cross 10,000 miles across two continents and arrive in the United States with two children, two bags, and a few hundred dollars.

Mine was a typical immigrant's story of reaching for safety for my children, mixed with my own big dreams, although I wondered how I would manage it with only knowing a few words in English. Maybe not so typical was the terror I felt when my son was kidnapped, or when I held a cold revolver in my shaking hand, facing masked men who'd been sent to my home to collect debts from my filthy rich Novo-Russian ex-husband. The fear I'd felt in that memory passed now as the power of the feeling of freedom I remember returned, and which I experienced for the first time when I landed on American soil. No more guns or threats to my children. I would do anything for that.

I didn't think about how I'd worked for $5 an hour in a shop selling antique furniture, and as a technician in a sperm bank, while studying to take the USMLE exam to get into the medical residency. I didn't remember the two or three jobs I worked at for decades to support my growing children, or the hurtful words from one of my colleagues that put me into tears.

The chest pain was lingering somewhere deep in my chest. *Let it be.* I wasn't scared. I felt happy and at home in the hospital. It wasn't a matter of what country I was in; the hospital was my home, and the nurses and doctors were "my people." For more than 30 years I had been one of them; I was a doctor.

That evening, my doctor's "compassion" muscle had got overworked. As it frequently happens to people speaking a foreign language, when emotions overflow, words do not come out in response. Instead, emotions bundle in the chest in a little ball. That "ball," for me, became alive and transformed into a bird, who spread its wings and painfully tried to find a place inside of my heart. My chest responded to its presence with shortened breaths, almost like it didn't want to disturb the struggling bird. That panicking bird didn't want to leave my chest till the next day, reminding me of its existence through the night. The consciousness of my clinician's mind sent warning signs: "chest pain on exertion and shortness of breath in the middle-aged woman." *Wake up, doctor!* I did not have an elephant sitting on my chest, as it's supposed to feel during a heart attack, I had a "little bird." *It's going to be okay.*

The medical assistant at my new primary care doctor's office, where I'd arrived early in the morning, was visibly irritated with me—a demanding patient—asking to have their blood pressure rechecked. "What did you say my blood pressure is? 190 over 100? It cannot be right." I eat healthily, jog 10 miles a week and do a headstand during my yoga practice. I reassure patients all the time that lifestyle modifications and stress management do work and should be tried before prescribing medications. The medical assistant looked at my electrocardiogram and clearly wanted to leave the room as quickly as possible.

"Can I take a peek?" I asked. I saw concern in his eyes. The familiar concave ST segment—the elevation pattern on the electrocardiogram of a classic heart attack—were signs that blood supply to my heart might be blocked. *It can't be happening to me!* I would rather believe that I had mysteriously developed vision and hearing impairments than trust that I might have heart disease.

"We have to call 911," my doctor said, almost apologetically.

Wait a minute, I'm the one who usually says *we have to call 911.* "No 911, please," I responded. I signed the "Against medical advice" papers, took a picture of my electrocardiogram and left.

Bright sun blinded me as I exited the office. I glimpsed back and met the concerned look of the receptionist. "I am gonna be fine!" I mouthed, hoping she could read my lips, as my habitual intention of making people around me feel better kicked in.

It seemed then that all my reasonable senses wanted to ignore my medical emergency and focus on the beauty around me instead:

bright sun, warm wind, and the smell of blooming orange trees. Positive thinking and holding on to anything that connects us with normalcy is a known defense mechanism against stress. *Life is good!* My doctor's judgment was "watching" me as a patient in an almost hypnotic state. What do we do when we're stressed? We eat. "Sushi," I said, as I saw the sign next door and walked into the restaurant.

Memory is a funny thing. *The Last Supper* fresco by Leonardo da Vinci, which I admired in the Santa Maria delle Grazie Dominican monastery in Milan, unexpectedly came to mind. It can't be my "last supper." If so, it's not bad! It's my favorite food! Will this tray of sushi betray me, like my efforts of almost daily exercise and a sinless diet? My weight and cholesterol were perfect, why would I have heart disease? Is it God's plan for me? I pictured again the apostles and Jesus, who, despite pain and suffering, gathered for the last meal, captured by Leonardo da Vinci.

Fortunately, the doctor in me interrupted my patient's philosophical reasoning and re-assessed the medical vignette: middle-aged female with acute onset of on-and-off chest pain and shortness of breath after a stressful event at work. Most likely anxiety. Then why is there highly elevated blood pressure and an abnormal electrocardiogram? This did not make a category of anxiety as a differential diagnosis. "Needs cardiac evaluation," was the *doctor's* assessment. I texted the picture of my EKG to my colleague cardiologist without saying that it belonged to me. When I'd finished my chai tea, he texted back: "Send your patient to the ER, I'll meet her there in 20 minutes."

I called an Uber and arrived at the emergency department. Twenty minutes later, after laboratory results had confirmed a high probability of my heart muscle being injured, I fell asleep staring at the ceiling of the cath lab, with the joyous thoughts of my adventurous life and feeling grateful to God for all the gifts I had received.

• • •

"I have good news and bad news," said my cardiologist when I woke up. The good news was that my faithful, healthy lifestyle had not betrayed me; proving once more that science is right. My coronary arteries were "clean as a whistle," and I hadn't had a heart attack. The bad news was that my *heart was broken*.

"Broken heart syndrome" or Takotsubo cardiomyopathy, is a medical term for a sudden weakening of the left ventricle—the heart's main pumping system—which can happen as a result of severe emotional (more common in women) or physical (more frequent in men) stress. I was happy with the verdict as it meant I didn't have to have any procedures or surgeries. The funny word, "Takotsubo," didn't mean much to me at that moment. It comes from the Japanese *takotsubo* or "octopus pot" and was given to this condition by Japanese physician Hikaru Sato, from Hiroshima City Hospital, who first recognized reversible left ventricular apical wall motion abnormalities that were often associated with emotional or physical stress and frequently affected women over 50.[1]

The history of broken heart syndrome goes back more than three decades. In 1986, a 44-year-old woman was admitted to Massachusetts General Hospital with severe chest pain after learning about her son's suicide. Her coronary arteries were clear of blockages or narrowing.[2] The mother's heart had literally "broken" from the wealth of emotions and grief, which had caused a weakening of the heart muscle.

The chest pain, shortness of breath, electrocardiogram and blood test changes that patients with Takotsubo cardiomyopathy experience are similar to a classic heart attack. The main difference is that plaques in the coronary vessels and dependent myocardial changes, typical of a myocardial infarction, are usually absent in patients with Takotsubo. *Broken heart syndrome* results from the enormous release of catecholamines (hormones), provoked by the activation of the autonomic nervous and neuroendocrine systems during stressful events. Activation of the hypothalamic–pituitary–adrenal axis and the release of corticotropin-releasing hormone (CRH) stimulates epinephrine and a norepinephrine release by the adrenal glands, as well as norepinephrine release from the sympathetic nerve endings. These catecholamines stimulate cardiovascular and respiratory responses of rising blood pressure, heartrate and breathing rate, in addition to muscle tension. Redirecting the blood flow arouses the brain and prepares the muscles and the heart for a "fight or flight" response. Catecholamines also stimulate blood cell activation, leading to temporary clotting of small vessels, which is another physiological response to not bleed during the "fight."[3]

Although life-threatening complications in the acute phase can cause death in one to eight people out of 100 cases,[4] the changes in the hearts of Takotsubo cardiomyopathy patients are reversible, and "broken hearts" can heal. The real problem with this mysterious illness is that there is no well-proven cure or reliable treatment for it. Multiple causes have been considered as a potential explanation, with inflammation recognized to be a fundamental part of the pathophysiology, but the cause–effect relationship remains unknown.[5] As a primary care doctor, I haven't had patients with this diagnosis, and I knew that research on the treatments was quite elusive.

• • •

I left the hospital with a prescription for a beta-blocker—medication to improve my heart's pumping function, control blood pressure and oppose the actions of catecholamines—and a recommendation to control my stress, the major trigger. A few months later, I started feeling more drained and tired, with occasional dizzy spells and nightmares, which were medication side effects I often warned my patients about, always adding that it's worth it because the beta-blockers prolong the life of patients with heart disease. To improve my heart function, I had to exercise, but the beta-blocker made my fatigue too big an obstacle for my habitual physical activity.

Here I was, after 35 years of practice and thousands of patients healed, feeling lost, so how did my patients feel in this situation? It was a skin-crawling experience.

I am a firm believer that there is a purpose in every challenge God sends us. We just have to discover it. Being in the patient's shoes is an experience that we, as doctors, should endure sometimes. I have advised probably thousands of patients about controlling their stress. So, *what should I actually be doing?* I wondered. Well-known stress-relief strategies are regular exercise, mindfulness, and healthy eating habits. They did not help me. I felt betrayed by my own body, and I lost faith in what I'd been preaching to my patients every day. The stress was exponentially growing, in fact.

"When the patient's voice is heard and considered, a better solution emerges," I was teaching my residents, encouraging them to listen to patients' stories and their own attitude toward malady. What was my voice telling me now? Scientific reviews about Takotsubo cardiomyopathy advise that "treatments should be decided on an individual basis, with careful consideration of the risks and benefits involved."[6] If stress reduction was the advice, I had to figure out what triggered my stressful reactions and what had worked for me in the past. What else was out there to conquer that stress? Are there any other remedies that have the same benefits as beta-blockers on the heart without the side effects? I started my own search for answers, as many of my patients do.

"Don't be upset with me, but I found this information and decided…" I often heard my patients say. People feel guilty and apologize for questioning doctors' opinions and looking for alternative treatment options. But no apologies are necessary! That's what *partners* do—provide constructive feedback and collaborate in seeking knowledge to get the best outcome. So, how can you be effective in your communication with your clinician? Let's look into this.

PART ONE

LEARN ABOUT YOURSELF

"Knowing yourself is the beginning of all wisdom."

ARISTOTLE

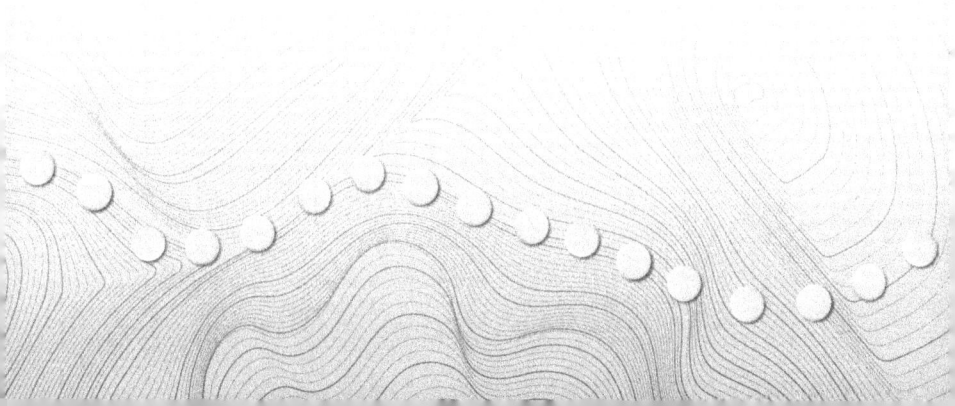

CHAPTER 1

DO YOUR PART

grew up in a place that is not for "wimps!" Siberia, an area of Russia that extends from the Ural Mountains in the west to the Pacific
Ocean in the east, north to Kazakhstan and the borders of China.
When I talk about Siberia, people imagine bears walking in the snow,
and taiga forests interrupted by headwaters of powerful rivers, which
is far from reality. Because of notorious wars and threats to Russia,
and the need to preserve and protect the country's industry, academic
and scientific resources, Siberia has transformed from the land with
the name *Tatar*—meaning "sleeping land"—and place of exile for
criminals and political and war prisoners, to the center of science in
chemistry, physics, information technologies, and medicine.

Factories and academic institutions were evacuated from Central
Russia at the time of World War II and were rebuilt and populated
with the brilliant minds of former political and war prisoners from
the camps spread throughout Siberian land. European culture and
education were tightly mixed with the Asian roots of the local com-
munities. The city of Tomsk, where I graduated from medical school,
is one of the oldest towns in Siberia. It harbors six state universities,
over 120,000 students, and five scientific medical centers. Not what
you'd expect from a Siberian town?

Tomsk is a city of half a million people, but it wasn't on the world maps till the late '80s, being one of the "closed to foreigners" cities. One had to pass checkpoints to show entry documents. There was a true secret town too, known as "Tomsk-7," later renamed Seversk, nine miles northwest of Tomsk, and it became home to the Sibirskaya Nuclear Power Plant, one of the Soviet Union's first industrial-scale nuclear power stations. I don't think it's a coincidence that the National Research Medical Center, with centers for medical genetics, oncology, cardiology, obstetrics, gynecology and perinatology, pharmacology, and regenerative medicine research were built next to the nuclear plant. It merged science with technology infrastructure, which all started from the medical patriarch, Siberian State Medical University, my alma mater. However, the real spirit of Siberia is reflected by the toughness, independence, and commonsense of the rural people, molded by the harsh environment they live in.

My mother was a surgeon in the faculty of the Siberian State Medical University. When I was a kid, almost every summer I spent time on a small ship with my mother and other medical university faculty colleagues traveling more than 2,000 miles of the River Ob to rural villages, where people didn't have access to healthcare during the heavy Siberian winters. The ship was a mini hospital with fully equipped operating rooms and tiny exam rooms, where faculty, residents, medical students, and nursing staff examined and treated patients, performed surgeries and procedures. Most of the healthcare in rural towns and villages was provided by "feldshers," medical professionals with one year of medical education, with few physicians. The six feet of snow in the forests during winter, plus frozen rivers without bridges, were significant barriers for farmers and their families who lived there. Helicopters were available for transport of trauma victims, surgical, and complicated labor and deliveries.

Together with other children of physicians and medical staff, we cleaned and stocked patients' rooms, filled up the huge samovar for tea, and helped with signing up patients. It was our responsibility to entertain the patients who were waiting to be seen or operated-on. We read poems by heart, sang and danced, doing whatever it took to make people smile. Grateful patients used to bring delicious homecooked food, pickled vegetables, mushrooms, honey, and wild berries.

One evening, when my mother returned after ten hours in the operating room, exhausted but happy, I asked a question that bothered me. "How do all these people live separated by hundreds of miles of snow the whole year without seeing doctors?"

My mother looked at me with a heartening smile. "They take charge of their health—they eat right, don't eat a lot, mostly natural, healthy food, wild berries, mushrooms and a lot of herbs. They know simple, natural remedies for colds, cuts, and bruises. They do a lot of physical work. If something happens, and they need urgent, complicated procedures or operations, feldshers ship them by helicopter to the nearest hospital. We will do the rest in the summer."

In my current understanding of medicine, this translates to principles of self-care, healthy nutrition combined with an active lifestyle, and accessible triage for sick patients. Doctors trust patients' commonsense and their ability to recognize dangerous medical conditions and seek help when necessary.

Do we go to the doctor as soon as we feel a sore throat, backache, stuffy nose, stomachache, diarrhea or are just feeling down and tired? The first steps of medical care we make ourselves. Sometimes we wait and see, hoping nature will take its course or we ask advice from family and friends. We might consult Dr. Google, which has become an instant medical advisor for many. We make our own medical decisions and seek help online, from doctors' offices, urgent care or the emergency room. Clinicians can only solve our medical problems if we reach out to them, tell our story and ask for help.

If you think doctors know the answers to every medical dilemma patients come in with, it's absolutely not the case. Doctors are professionals, though, who know how human bodies work; they are familiar with the diseases that are out there and are skilled in using diagnostic algorithms and treating illnesses. Pulling out a single piece of knowledge—the sign or symptom—is only useful when doctors learn your story, examine your body for signs of suspected illness, and clarify raised uncertainties by using different tests. Doctors need YOU to guide them in the decisions they make.

"I am your partner in crime, as long as we don't commit too much crime!" I often tell my patients. "Why do you think we would commit a crime?" asked Robert Hanger, a delightful farmer from Walterboro, a small town in South Carolina, who agreed with my every suggestion until we started talking about insulin to treat his advanced diabetes. Despite his high blood glucose numbers, Robert refused to take insulin, which would have been the best choice for his diabetes based on the known evidence-based guidelines at that time, before we had new, more powerful diabetes medications. "That is not the best choice for me," said Robert, acknowledging ownership of his health journey.

Physicians may agree with a patient's choice without asking why, and let the patient miss the opportunity to get the best treatment. When there is an established trust between a patient and a doctor, patients are more likely to disclose their reasons. "Tell me what to do and I'll do it, but I can't see myself being on insulin. My father was only 60 when he died, ten years after he started taking insulin." Robert shook his head, clearly not ready to follow my "evidence-based" guidelines.

"Insulin is not the best choice for me," he said, fully accepting his leading role. We postponed insulin treatment and he agreed to try other medications and lifestyle changes. We also allocated times to assess his progress. He became much more invested in his life-style-changing efforts and won his battle with diabetes faster than I thought he would.

BE AN ACTIVE PATIENT

The word "patient" comes from the Latin *patiens*, from *patior*, to suffer or bear. In my opinion, the word "patient" must be put to rest for many reasons. Suffering is not always necessary anymore for those who come to see a doctor. The time has passed when patients granted complete decision-making power to physicians, seldom questioning their authority. It's almost impossible anymore to see the typical Talcott Parsons' "sick role" of passive patients who "put themselves into the hands" of "competent" physicians, surrendering responsibility and control of their health. The *active patient* concept has grown gradually within the last two centuries following societal interest toward autonomy and personal responsibility.[7] These days, patients, with Dr. Google on their side, and equipped with their medical records and free access to online educational resources, not only ask sophisticated questions but also doubt doctors' recommendations.

Many modern "patients" are actually doing well; they want to live longer lives while practicing "wellness," making informed choices about lifestyle, fertility and cosmetic surgery, and reaching out to physicians for advice. Most importantly, many of us don't like to be "patients." Do you? The word itself brings feelings of vulnerability and a stamp of "illness."

The word "doctor" comes from the Latin word for teacher, meaning "to teach."[8] *Vrach* in Russian, *artz* in German, *médico* in Spanish, *lékař* in Czech, *dokter* in Dutch; doctors teach others how to be healthy, and diagnose and treat illnesses. A redistribution of power between patients and physicians in health oversight, or sharing a doctor's role, has already been going on. Instead of the image of suffering, and grateful patients, the relationship between a doctor and a patient has become one of equals.[9] Without realizing, patients have already become their own doctors through sharing decisions about diagnostic workup and treatment options with physicians.

I have worked with, learned from, and taught hundreds of talented, knowledgeable expert-clinicians, which has helped me realize that being a patient of the most knowledgeable and competent physician will not assure my health and wellbeing. Principles of self-reliance, commonsense, lifelong learning and a mindfully created community of health advisors, including medical professionals, will.

Modern technology has opened the doors of online medical communication, access to personal medical information—doctors' notes, laboratory tests and imaging—as well as a library of endless information on the internet. But do you know how to use it to your advantage? Are you asking questions? Are you asking questions on time—when physicians make decisions about your treatment? Are you telling your doctor what treatment you can't accept for one reason or another; financially because of your busy lifestyle, or, simply, because you are not ready yet? These and many other questions about learning self-reliance and mindful medical self-care will be answered in the following chapters.

"Why do I have to know that?" You may ask.

Because you don't want to silently accept what is offered by a doctor without expressing your life circumstances, barriers and perceptions. Doctors need detailed information to make a diagnosis, which only you or your family can provide. Being a partner entitles you to present your point of view, to give your clinician a chance to offer you the best option that would fit your life. Some might say, "Doctors don't like patients who argue with their decisions." Yet physicians learn and build their expertise not only on the scientific facts, but on patients' feedback and responses to treatment. While communicating your point of view about your illness and related aspects of your life, you will learn the best ways to present opinions in an organized and timely fashion.

I also hear a lot, "My doctor isn't interested in my opinion." Time pressures have become an overwhelming barrier that has made the patient-doctor relationship challenging. Medicine is a business, after all, that requires doctors to see more patients. During the allotted time for a patient's visit, doctors not only listen to the patient, examine them, and come up with the diagnosis and treatment; they also place orders for tests and make referrals so that your treatment can get started. This is not an excuse, but an invitation for a patient-doctor partnership. "It takes two to tango." Do your part!

CHECK YOUR HEALTHCARE INVENTORY:

1. Write down the facts of your medical history: diagnosed illnesses, family history, surgeries, medication list, allergies.

2. Keep paper or electronic files of your previous testing/ procedures (recent mammogram, colonoscopy, stress test, echocardiogram, or other diagnostic procedures). Collect the information and have it ready to bring with you for the first visit with a doctor.

3. After the doctor's visit, log in to your "electronic medical records (EMR) Patient Portal and verify if the medical information there is correct.

CHAPTER 2

RISKS AND HEALTH MAP

Risk" is one of the most commonly used words in health-related headlines. It tells about our exposure to danger or potential losses.[10] Doctors estimate patients' risk factors to learn about their chances of developing illnesses, and to focus on prevention or anticipate complications of existing illnesses to intensify the treatments. Many diseases have been conquered at the population level by reducing hazards and controlling the environment, water supply, the air we breathe, and offering immunizations. But two-thirds of deaths globally lie on our own responsibility for the risks brought about by our lifestyle choices: obesity, smoking, injuries, and stress.[11] Some of the risk factors cannot be modified, such as your age, ethnicity, or genetic history. Others are within your control, such as your lifestyle, habits, occupation, and whether you wear a seatbelt in the car or a helmet on your bike.

The good news about risks is that many of them can be controlled; diseases can be prevented, caught earlier, and treatment started before complications happen. Understanding the value of health risks is similar to planning a road trip and having a road map. Write down your habits, existing and potential risks, and try to make connections between them. Then add diseases that you've been diagnosed with and draw connections (lines) toward your habits and risks. That's your health map. The map is a symbolic representation of landmarks and routes, which help us to avoid dangerous areas and figure out the most effective path from one point to another. You may skip traveling through rural Montana during the winter, for example, if you have a small car and don't want to invest in warm clothes and winter tires! Similarly, if you have a risk of premature heart disease, you may invest in a healthy lifestyle, stop smoking, and pay attention to your weight and activity levels.

Knowing your habits and risk factors gives you an insight into the likelihood of cancer, heart disease, autoimmune disorders, asthma, depression, and many others. It also helps you to make decisions about health driven by facts and not fears. Chest pain in someone who smoked and has a family history of premature heart disease must be treated differently and with much more caution than chest pain in someone who doesn't have those risks. More frequent colonoscopies are necessary when you have a history of polyps, or more aggressive cholesterol management to reduce your risk of heart disease.

HOW DO DOCTORS DETERMINE PATIENTS' HEALTH RISKS?

Doctors look at risks associated with age and gender,[12] family history, environment, and what we know about harmful ramifications of smoking, alcohol consumption, overeating, and risky behaviors of drug misuse and "unsafe" sex. The risks of childhood and adolescent diseases historically depend on the socio-demographic index (SDI)—a composite indicator of income, educational attainment, and fertility. We, as parents, can influence the health of our children by following physicians' recommendations during regular prenatal visits and pediatric checkups, following age-based immunizations and safety precautions.

Knowledge of a patient's place of long-term residence or work can also help place risk and aid early diagnosis. For example, I knew that

Tim Baker was an IT engineer. He came in for the onset of headaches and thought that these were related to stress at work, and long hours spent in front of the computer screen. He focused on stress-relieving techniques such as yoga, meditation, and good sleep. Tim's headaches sounded like migraine—one sided, pulsating, with some nausea and visual changes—until his wife called to say that Tim was in the emergency department with a seizure.

A brain MRI showed two neurocysticercosis brain cysts; sacs containing the immature stage of a parasitic tapeworm. After people have eaten food contaminated with tapeworm, secretions in the stomach cause the eggs to hatch into larvae. The larvae enter the bloodstream and can spread to different parts of the body, including the brain and spinal cord, where the larvae form cysts. These cysts cause few symptoms until the cysts degenerate and the larvae die, triggering inflammation, swelling and symptoms, such as headaches, seizures, personality changes, and mental impairment.[13] Knowing that he had traveled to a third-world country, which was followed by a new onset of headache, prompted the order of a brain MRI or CT scan in the first place.

McKenzie West was seen in the ER for abdominal pain. The CT scan of her abdomen showed a 2cm pulmonary nodule in the base of her left lung. Incidental findings of pulmonary nodules are a common source of reasonable anxiety, especially when the nodules are larger than 5mm. Thoughts about lung cancer and metastatic disease from undiscovered cancer kept her awake at night. A test for coccidioidomycosis, performed as part of the work up, showed the presence of Valley Fever, a common fungal disease. The Coccidioides fungus is known to live in the soil in the southwestern United States, central Washington, parts of Mexico, and Central and South America. People get Valley Fever by breathing in the fungal spores from the air. Most people don't even know about this illness because they don't feel sick. Those who get sick usually get better on their own within weeks to months. Only a few will require antifungal treatment.[14] Knowledge of residence can help diagnose common fungal infections and sequelae of them can guide the testing.

When Dan Rogers showed up with a cough and chest pain, symptoms for a common cold, Dr. Cohen was rightfully concerned about a blood clot in his lung, which was confirmed on the lung images within an hour. Dan was a pilot who had just returned from a long trip to Thailand. Long trips by air or car can increase the risk for blood-clot formation in the large veins, which are reported in up to 10 percent of passengers on long-haul flights.[15] Blood clots or their parts may break off and travel to the lungs, causing a sudden blockage of arteries in the lung, known as a pulmonary embolism (PE). Letting the doctor know about the travel you've done when you're experiencing leg swelling or chest pain with shortness of breath might be lifesaving.

Doctors can overestimate or underestimate the dangers if patients don't rationally think about them and communicate to the clinician. When risks are known, there is always an option to be passive and leave the odds to luck.

Breast cancer killed my mother at the age of 46, so I thought this would be my unfortunate "constitutional" bad luck too. In an attempt to take control of my destiny, I explored my "risk" for breast cancer by using risk calculators and getting BRCA testing. Surprisingly, I felt *disappointed* when I received a negative on genetic BRCA testing. If it was positive, I had a plan of action to have my breasts and ovaries removed and monitor my pancreas every year. But it was negative. I was back to where I was before with uncertainty about my five-year risk for breast cancer, being five times higher than women of the same race and age.

As the American anthropologist Steve Rayner pointed out, uncertainty is the gray area between the darkness of ignorance (or the absence of knowledge) and the light of certainty (or the presence of demonstrated knowledge).[16] Certainty gives more peace of mind to some, but pointless worry to others. I did not like to worry, so opted to get peace from yearly mammograms. I also refused hormone replacement therapy, even when the hot flashes of early menopause became unbearable. Do we always think rationally about risks and make judgments that are expected to reduce them? In many ways, our perception of risk is irrational and often superstitious. Some people find the discussion about health risks intimidating. "The less I think about it, the less chance it's going to happen."

RISKS ILLUSIONS

The most common and powerful reason why we do not want to accept our risks is a phenomenon known as "positive illusions." According to research, most people overestimate their health or lifespan, sometimes by more than 20 years, and underestimate the likelihood of cancer or cardiovascular events. There is a high level of confidence present in most of us that our life will be better and last longer than our peers.[17] This thought process is known as optimism bias. The brain plays a trick that boosts positive illusions, especially about our future.

Dr. Tali Sharot, a neuroscientist, demonstrated in her book, *The Optimism Bias: A Tour of the Irrationally Positive Brain*, that optimism is crucial to human existence.[18] About 80 percent of us, according to most estimates, display an optimism bias that was observed across gender, race, nationality and age. From as early as 18 years old until age 80, we are not inclined to see ourselves going through poor health, financial insecurity, divorces, professional failures, and other unhappy events. We wear rose-tinted glasses at ages 60 to 80 just as much as at ages 18 to 25.

People often find experts' opinions on health risks confusing, and government and media sources untrustworthy. Personal beliefs and experience, as well as the expertise of people we trust, are more pivotal factors in decision-making for many. In relationships with the risk factors, we express four types of behaviors:

1. Followers
2. Optimists
3. Dogmatics
4. Indifferent

Followers unquestionably trust the opinions of doctors who are shown to have knowledge and expertise in the field, whether on paper or by their personal experience. It's hard to convince followers to stop medication that was prescribed by the "expert doctor" or stop unnecessary Pap smears. They also don't participate in shared decision-making, by avoiding bringing up their own experiences and beliefs.

Optimists always hope for the best and don't want to contemplate the worst. "We haven't had colon cancer in the family. I feel good. I don't want any screenings." They question the diagnosis, which could not or should not happen. They ignore offered screenings and increase their risks of preventable diseases.

Dogmatics have their own point of view on medical problems and stick to them, often without explanation. "I don't do immunizations; they change my genes." "I will only take natural products." Depending on their beliefs, doctors may not be aware of what supplements or other interventions these people take in addition to prescribed treatments and may agree to order unnecessary tests under pressure.

The last category is those who are *indifferent* to the outcomes. "I don't care." "Whatever!" Clinicians never know if they will do the procedure or ordered test or whether they will take the medication. They don't have a point of view on an issue. For one reason or another, they generally don't care about their future and feel comfortable with the serendipity of illness. I frequently see this approach in teenagers.

Who are you? Can you identify yourself with any of these categories?

Each limits the chances for a rational estimate of your risks and therefore determines the path you are going to take in your health journey. Will your negative attitude towards immunizations play a role in the development of severe symptoms and potential death instead of having a light form of illness? If your indifferent attitude toward your future is something you can accept, and you can live in peace with late diagnosis of illness, then let it be. You choose the route on your health map.

The nature of risk also plays a role in how we respond to it.[19] Habitually, we overestimate the likelihood of low-probability/high-consequence risks (such as being injured or killed by a tornado or in a plane crash), and we tend to underestimate the risk of harm from more common and dangerous causes, such as high blood pressure or diabetes. We are more sensitive to a risk if it is involuntary, inescapable, poorly understood by science, or subject to contradictory statements.[20] Instead of guessing and living in fear, or resisting the knowledge and doing nothing, we would be much safer to calculate a risk's probability and "margins for safety" to estimate the most reasonable individual approaches for prevention. There are many risk calculators online. But are these risk-assessment instruments/calculators/apps online good resources to estimate the risk for heart disease, cancer, osteoporosis, etc.? There are three problems with them:

1. Not all calculators found online or in app stores are validated—they only give a ballpark guess about your level of risk.

2. Not everyone knows how to interpret the results correctly.

3. Risk calculators are only as good as the information you enter. If you enter your test result—for example, your blood pressure or cholesterol—incorrectly or from last year, the risk score will be off.

As patients, we tend to perceive ambiguity as a threat and focus on creating certainty. Will partial or unvalidated facts fill the blanks of our future and be worthy of acting on them? False certainty is an illusion. Instead, invest in validated assessments, bring doctors' expertise in to weigh the risks and discuss prevention, and definitely don't defer it. A lot of my patients schedule preventive wellness visits after their birthday to discuss their risks—old ones and new ones—and plan preventive strategies for the year ahead. Plan your health journey ahead and look at your health map as an investment in the future that always pays off.

CHECK YOUR HEALTHCARE INVENTORY:

1. What do you think your health risks are? Write down the three risk factors you think are the most relevant for your future.

2. Go to the US Preventative Task Force website and compare your estimate with preventive recommendations based on your risks and gender. What are the differences?

3. If you have not had a wellness exam, visit your doctor to discuss your health risks.

CHAPTER 3

GENETIC LOAD

With curly dark hair and dark brown eyes behind round glasses, Jarrad Roswald had the nerdy look of a smart kid. He'd grown up in a prominent Jewish family in New York City and held a PhD in chemistry. He scheduled physicals every year "to make sure I'm okay." His physical exams were normal as well as his cholesterol and blood glucose. Shy and introverted, he did not like playing sports as a child. There was a family stigma, that "things could happen," "better be careful." His mother seemed to "not feel well" most of her life and died from breast cancer in her early 50s. His father was too busy with his job in the bank and died from a heart attack after yet another late meeting.

Jarrad had decided that he didn't want to live like his parents. From his college years he exercised regularly, became a vegetarian, and spent a lot of time outdoors. When he graduated from Princeton, he moved from New York City to Charleston, SC, known for its relaxing beach-town lifestyle. Last spring, Jarrad had a beautiful southern wedding at the Magnolia Plantation. Now, he and his wife were eager to start a family. After I gave him a clean bill of health, he pulled out a stack of colorful papers with DNA testing reports. These recognized his Ashkenazi Jewish ancestry and an increased risk for several diseases, including breast cancer and thrombophilia.

"What should I do about this?" he asked. "My wife is pregnant. I'm terrified that our child will be sick. I'm scared to even show these reports to her."

Genetic or DNA testing examines genes, chromosomes, or proteins to identify changes or variations (mutations), which can cause or increase the risk of a genetic disorder. DNA testing popularity has exploded since the mapping of the human genome in 2003. In 2017 there were approximately 75,000 genetic tests on the market, representing approximately 10,000 unique test types, with about ten new tests entering the market daily.[21] It became a multimillion-dollar industry driven by consumers wondering about their roots and potentially extending their life based on genetic information.

I understood his worries. When both my adult children bought 23andMe testing kits, I was more nervous than they were. I might be the one to blame for "bad genetics." I remembered my own thoughts when I turned 46—the same age as my mother when she died from breast cancer—and being overwhelmed with the expectancy of illness that might never be cured and would only die with me. "Should I get my bucket list filled?" was my question that year.

I went through the memories of both my pregnancies while a young physician in Siberia. The lengthy working hours, sleepless nights on call, and the never-ending stress of worrying about my babies and my patients, which could surely break even healthy "genetic codes." Pregnant women who work long hours with high levels of psychological stress belong to the high obstetrical risk group. The adverse pregnancy outcomes may occur through a mechanism related to increased levels of stress hormones and standing up for long hours that make changes in uterine blood flow.[22] Both my mother and I, as practicing physicians, belonged in that group. As my mother had, I continued doing surgeries while pregnant with both of my children, in operating rooms with half-open ether systems; a pleasant smell but hazardous chemicals used in Russia back then for patients' general anesthesia. Patients experienced that anesthesia once during the surgery, but surgeons were exposed to it day after day with every patient. Life in Siberia next to the nuclear reactor could have been the match that struck my genetic load on fire.

While my children were excited to know their "ancestry traits," I went straight to their health genetic risks, looking for evidence of "being guilty" in my selfishness. Selfishly loving my profession, living in a town in Siberia where radiation exposure from the nuclear reactor was higher than average, and many other risky, stupid things I probably did back then. The working-mom guilt quickly kicked in. Fortunately for my family, their DNA reports didn't reveal any genetic variants that may affect their health, and the tests were quickly forgotten. That was a relief! But I decided not to do genetic testing for myself, accepting an old-fashioned level of uncertainty, rather than facing the certainty of dealing with the risk of illness.

Jarrad's grandparents had immigrated from Lithuania—the country he always wanted to visit one day. Ashkenazi (Ashkenazi meaning "German" in Hebrew) Jews were studied more than any other population for medical and population genetics because of the long-standing "purity" of the group among others.[23] One in five Ashkenazi Jews carry a mutation for the genetic disorders cystic fibrosis, Canavan disease, familial dysautonomia, Tay-Sachs disease, Fanconi anemia, Niemann-Pick disease, Bloom syndrome, mucolipidosis IV, and Gaucher disease.[24] Ashkenazi Jews have been found to have specific gene mutations that increase their susceptibility to certain forms of cancers. Mutations in both breast cancer genes (BRCA1 and BRCA2) were found in one out of 40 Ashkenazi Jewish women, increasing their likelihood of breast or ovarian cancer. Ashkenazi Jews have the highest lifetime risk of colorectal cancer among any ethnic group in the world, almost twice higher than non-Ashkenazi populations (9–15 percent). Pancreatic cancer, carcinomas of the stomach and non-Hodgkin lymphoma have a higher incidence among the Ashkenazi population too.[25]

Prenatal (during pregnancy) genetic testing and hereditary cancer tests account for the highest percentage of conventional genetic testing ordered by physicians, followed by oncology genetic diagnostics and treatment testing.[26] Everyone who reports the presence of certain diseases in multiple family members has the option to get consultation from genetic specialists and comprehensive genetic testing. Some prefer the option of commercial DNA testing, which is a more widespread "shotgun" approach, than a targeted approach advised by a genetic counselor. Commercial direct-to-consumer (DTC) DNA testing doesn't intend to diagnose diseases but delivers a lot of engaging information about ancestry, health predisposition to complex diseases, such as hereditary cancers, cardiovascular disease and depression, and pharmacogenetics (potential reactions to certain medications) and carrier state.

ARE THE TESTS VALID?

After the initial excitement of finding new relatives on other continents, people often ask questions about the validity and privacy of the tests. Patients come to their primary care physician (PCP) asking them to interpret the results and answer their questions: *Are these risks real? What should I do now?*

When patients ask for advice based on the test, doctors have to determine, first, how reliable any test is before drawing recommendations. When physicians order any test, they expect accuracy. They send specimens to the laboratories where health-related tests are subject to federal regulatory standards. The Food and Drug Administration (FDA) requires information about clinical validity for only some genetic tests. Most health predisposition reports include *genetic likelihood* based on the company's *own genetic research model* from former customers' results, which might not be relevant for all consumers.[27] It's hard for doctors to make definite recommendations based on a test, particularly if the testing laboratory warning states that the test *"is not intended to tell you anything about your current state of health, or to be used to make medical decisions, including whether or not you should take a medication, how much of a medication you should take, or determine any treatment."*[28]

So, how helpful can commercial DNA tests be? First, the results might make you less worried about getting a certain genetic disease. They can help doctors make recommendations about treatment or prevention of disease. This could be accomplished with the help of genetic counselors, who may repeat and verify conclusions of commercial DNA tests. You might be prompted to make lifestyle changes or seek help if you're found to be at risk for a certain disease. You may decide to be screened for diseases you are at risk of earlier or more often. A test could help your decision about having children and identifying genetic disorders early in life so treatment can be started as soon as possible.

There are some drawbacks you should be aware of too. DTC genetic testing often doesn't provide conclusive results on whether people will develop a disease or not. Diseases are influenced by environmental factors, age, sex, race, nutrition, exercise, and stress in addition to genetic factors. If you are affected by favorable environmental factors and have good nutrition and an active lifestyle, you might not develop the disease, despite a high genetic risk. On the contrary, someone with a low genetic risk may become sick if they live in a disease-prone environment or have lifestyle factors that increase susceptibility to the disease.[29] You might feel angry, anxious or depressed after getting the results, especially if you are diagnosed with an illness that does not have effective treatments. You might feel guilty, which could pass harm from the personal and professional choices you make to your family, as I did when my children decided to get testing. Commercial DNA testing involves significant cost, and your health insurance may not cover it or may only cover part of the cost.[30] It's up to you to make decisions based on the DTC results, which still might not be completely accurate, poorly related to you or non-deterministic.

WHAT ABOUT YOUR PRIVACY?

There is another aspect of commercial DNA testing that involves the privacy of your genetic code. "First rule of data: once you hand it over, you lose control of it. You have no idea how the terms of service will change for your 'recreational' DNA sample," tweeted Elizabeth Joh, a law professor at the University of California, Davis. Some of the biggest ancestry companies are owned in part by pharmaceutical giants or data companies—meaning your personal DNA information may be handed over to corporations to turn a profit. The data from consumers' genetic tests can be collected into databases to help with research in related fields, which you did not want to be part of but did not think about while signing the consent prior to the test.

It's easy to miss the "informed consent research" clauses. Informed consent gives the research participant information about how their personal information or specimen will be used for research purposes. When someone provides detailed information about themselves to find out more about their roots, they might not realize that their data is being used in genetic research, even though that information might be mentioned somewhere in the small print. Ancestry.com is owned, in part, by AOL and Compaq, both large data companies, as well as GIC—the Government of Singapore Investment Corporation—meaning Ancestry customers' DNA data belongs in part to a foreign government.[31]

Even when companies promise that they won't let the police into their databases without a warrant, it doesn't mean that they won't change their minds. According to the MIT Technology Review, Family Tree DNA allowed the FBI to upload DNA from corpses or blood spatters, and surf the database of about two million customers of the service, just like any other customer trying to locate and contact relatives.[32]

I reassured Jarrad that prenatal genetic screening programs are done routinely for pregnant women and referred him and his wife to a genetic specialist. It was a relief to find that he wasn't found to be a carrier for any of the mutations mentioned in the commercial DNA testing report. Two of his children became patients of our Family Medicine Center and, as with Jarrad, they never missed their health screening appointments.

With all the benefits of knowing your genetic load, DNA testing should not be used as a substitute for seeing your doctor for cancer and heart disease screenings or counseling on genetic and lifestyle habits that could increase or decrease your risks. If DNA testing showed that you are not at risk for a certain disease, especially cancer, I don't think that means you should skip checkups and screenings. Questions you should be asking your doctor include, should I be seeing a genetic counselor if I'm concerned about the increased risk of an illness that has been seen in my close family or multiple family members? What can I do to prevent it?

CHECK YOUR HEALTHCARE INVENTORY:

1. Write down the list of medical problems your parents and siblings have been diagnosed with. If you are not aware of their health issues, ask.

2. Talk to your family members about other relatives with similar medical problems and write the information down.

3. Discuss your family history with your physician and ask if there is merit for a genetic consult or simply check out commercial DNA testing options.

CHAPTER 4

FOOTPRINTS OR NORMALCY PATTERNS

Sarah Oh, 67, was proud of her garden, which she tirelessly worked on. It gave her joy and purpose. She nurtured her orange, lemon, and grapefruit trees to pack boxes of citrus fruits and donate them to city shelters and food banks. Always on the go, she expressed more energy in every move than most people her age. But not this day.

"My back hurts," she started. "I know my body. I've had pains here and there, who doesn't have those? But this is different. It's dull, right in the back." She pointed at the right sacroiliac joint.

"I love my garden. Look at this picture." She proudly showed me pictures of a lavish courtyard with pink and white gardenias, camellias and a patch of purple, pink and orange wildflowers with rows of citrus trees next to a white picket fence. "I slowed down my activity, put some heat and ice on it, and took ibuprofen for two months. But the pain hasn't gone away. It wakes me up at night. The doctor in urgent care gave me medication that made me sleepy but didn't take the pain away. I also went for physical therapy. Four weeks later, the pain is even sharper, with every move I make. Yesterday, both my legs swelled. I'm tired. I feel that something is really wrong."

Sarah was right to go from one doctor who didn't believe that her symptoms were different from her usual aches and pains, to another, who would. Sarah's laboratory tests showed anemia, a low count of red blood cells. This condition makes people feel tired and exhausted. She also had signs of acute kidney injury, a condition where the kidneys suddenly lose the ability to filter waste products from your blood. That's why fluid was building up in her legs. Sarah's pelvis x-ray showed punched-out spots on the bone, called "lytic." The verdict was that her back pain was a symptom of multiple myeloma, which is a cancer of the plasma cells. Those white blood cells accumulated in the bone marrow and developed abnormal proteins in the blood, called "monoclonal," which damaged the bones, caused anemia, and harmed her kidneys. Sarah was right: "something was really wrong."

Learning about our body parts is a milestone for our two-year-old selves; we learn them naturally, with little explanation. From early childhood, our adaptive unconscious thinking, like a giant computer, processes the data coming from neurons, vessels, and other tissues in an efficient and sophisticated manner, creating patterns of recognition. Kids quickly figure out that their mouth is for eating, eyes are for seeing, and their faces brighten when they see their mother. We don't teach children to jump or cry when they hear a loud sound, they just do it. When something is wrong, painful or unpleasant, children recognize it and cry.

We process and remember the body's signals that come from different organs as patterns of recognition associated with generated emotions. They stay in the memory and are recognized in milliseconds if repeated. Our senses—vision, hearing, smell, touch and taste—are perfect diagnostic tools. They assure our feelings of wellbeing and make new sensations apparent.

We recognize changes in our body from subtle sensations of loss of appetite to feeling sick. We can see red spots on the skin and make a conclusion about a rash.

You don't need expensive studies to notice the difference between your usual "feeling well" and new sensations your body sends you. The skill of *listening to your body* is not only about recognizing patterns of normalcy and identifying new sensations but also about learning to trust your subconscious memory and the "little voice" of intuitive thinking. Is this something you can learn? We teach medical students to ask patients questions about their bodies and perform as many exams as possible to learn "normal" first before identifying "abnormal." Most likely you are already doing it subconsciously. To notice signs of illness, start with spotting how your body looks and feels every day. I call these "normalcy" patterns or *body footprints*. They change with time and are influenced by age, the environments we are in, our habits, illnesses, and treatments. Just as we identify our skin being tanned after a day at the beach and accept it as a new version of *normal* that we see in the mirror; we recognize changes to our vision or hearing when we age that become familiar with time, and identify a certain feeling in our joints, which we wake up with every morning or develop after a long walk. We talk to doctors, get reassured that those feelings are just a sign of change, and move on, identifying them as our own.

CREATING YOUR BODY FOOTPRINT

Imagine having a digital scanner that you move from your head to your toes, checking each organ on the way. How are you doing?

You can check while in the shower, in front of a mirror or meditating. "Hello, my body! Is anything new? Is there anything different?" Do this periodically as a ritual to create your body footprint, just as medical students learn to distinguish normal from abnormal by practicing repetition, checking the review of systems, and examining patients. By following learned normalcy patterns, experienced clinicians can pick up even small delineations from normal. You have only one patient to worry about—or maybe two or three if you're a mother, habitually "scanning" your children's bodies, and bringing concerns to pediatricians.

Let's try it out. Go to the mirror. The easiest way is to do this before you take a shower. Look at yourself—yes, without makeup. Remember the color of your skin, eyes, lips, tongue. Notice the areas under your eyes. Some of us have habitual dark circles under the eyes, or puffiness, redness, thickness of eyebrows, etc. Remember them. Look at every discoloration (changes in color), redness, birthmarks on your body. Pay attention to the shapes, lines, contours, and curves. This is your body, the only one that is with you from birth to your last day. Take a mental picture of it without criticism, just for the sake of remembering and for comparing the feelings that arise from each part.

Take a breath in and out through your nose, then through your mouth. Feel the air coming in and going out and remember the speed of every inhale and exhale that feels good. Remember the depth of your breath when you are relaxed. Most of the time we don't hear our heartbeat, but if you do feel it regularly, recognize it. Feel the taste in your mouth, move your tongue around, look at your teeth. Is there any pain or discomfort? If you have pain or discomfort in certain areas—neck, knees or hips—ask yourself if this is familiar, how long has it been there? Make a mental checklist of your bodily concerns and set a date to return and recheck the areas of concern. Almost as if your doctor has asked you to return in a couple of days, a week or two.

Be gentle and kind with your body. You owe it so much, and you are in charge of it. You are in control. What has happened to it is the result of your actions. Try not to have regrets or judgments. Repeat your body scan ritual regularly to remember and recognize your normalcy pattern and create a mental checklist by going systematically through the different parts. It takes approximately 60 days for any habit to develop, so, after that, hopefully your body scan has become a habit and you will be able to recognize delineations from your body footprints.

As soon as you notice something new, whether it's congestion, swelling, headache or a lump, recognize it, try to remember the pattern, as doctors do. What, where, when, how much, what is it associated with? Do your best to describe it. This is so you can monitor it for a change and, most importantly, bring it up for your clinician's judgment. The better you describe it, the easier it is to make a correct diagnosis and start treatment.

CHECK YOUR HEALTHCARE INVENTORY:

1. Remember any symptoms you have experienced recently: headache, congestion, spots on the skin, nausea, etc. Try to describe them. Here are some tips:

    - Start with the visual if the problem is visible (skin spot or rash): location, size, color.

    - Follow this by feelings associated with it (pain, numbness, nausea).

    - What are the patterns? Is it persistent or comes and goes? What makes it worse and what makes it better?

    - Notice the timing—when did it start, how frequently has it been happening and for how long?

2. Use this approach to tell your clinician about your symptoms.

CHAPTER 5

DROWNING IN INFORMATION

Victorian author Jerome K. Jerome described a journey of three men in the classic tale, *Three Men in a Boat*. They had been riding a wooden skiff up the River Thames to escape the stress of 19th-century life between Kingston and Oxford. One of them had knee pain and consulted a medical encyclopedia for his symptoms. To his surprise, he discovered that he had all kinds of maladies, from typhoid and cholera to diphtheria—everything except for prepatellar bursitis, or housemaid's knee, that he actually suffered from. He also talked to his friends, Harris and George, and found out they suffered from lethargy. In a comical form, this is a classic example of how medical information can be misleading in the minds of non-health professionals. Instead of an encyclopedia these days, we have unlimited information online that is free and available for us to search.

Researchers have conducted multiple studies to explore consumers' online health information-seeking behaviors.[33,34] The major motivator for people who sought health information online was because of prior interactions between themselves and health professionals. My initial reaction to this was: are we, as clinicians, pushing our patients to look online instead? Is it a lack of trust, and our patients must verify our knowledge and the advice they've received?

Dr. Watson, who finished his residency two years ago, had a different opinion: "It doesn't matter why people search for health information. This is great if we engage patients' interest in health!" We were both right. People feel empowered and engaged in their medical care,[35,36] and are also driven by a lack of information provided by health professionals,[37,38] as well as dissatisfaction with their healthcare experiences.[39]

What do we look for online? Typically, it's information about medicines and medical devices, medical conditions, lifestyle information (diet and exercise), individual healthcare professionals, natural products, disease-specific associations, and the meaning of medical terms.

People also want to know more about what the doctor mentioned during their visit. Patients sometimes disagree with the doctor's opinion and seek confirmation online, as well as alternative options. Patients look for the emotional support of others with the same condition. There is a thinking that, *Maybe the doctor didn't tell me everything.*

"I start off with Google and see where that takes me." I've heard this from many of my patients. We go to forums and support groups to decide whether to purchase/use medications or natural products. Wikipedia is used as a resource for a trial of lifestyle intervention. Two-thirds of consumers obtain information from commercial websites, only little more than 11 percent use certain search engines and academically affiliated sites, and only about 5 percent use government-sponsored websites.[40] When I typed the word "diet" in a Google search, it returned 998,000,000 results in 0.61 seconds. The first four sources were sponsored advertisements, followed by Wikipedia, web media giants such as Healthline and WebMD, and five more pages of information that, on face value, seemed relevant to my search. Having so many choices is confusing and time consuming to explore.

WHAT INFORMATION WOULD
I LIKE MY PATIENTS TO HAVE?

Clinical information has to be reliable, up-to-date, free, accurate, easy to obtain, read and understand, and relevant to the person's issue. Let me share my go-to steps for an effective health information internet search.

1. Be specific when defining your question

This will save you a lot of time and effort. If you are looking for treatment, use "treatment of rheumatoid arthritis," not just "arthritis." Want to know how to diagnose heart failure? Use "diagnosis of heart failure." If you are looking for a single symptom, start with one word, for example "vomiting." When multiple websites come up, hold your initial reaction to click on the first one. The first websites are usually sponsored advertisements and are not always reliable. You can recognize them by the letters "Ad" at the front. The internet is a marketplace. Businesses pay for their websites to appear at the top of the search, to increase traffic to their sites. Businesses build successful marketing strategies around search engine optimization (SEO).

2. Be careful with symptom checkers

One symptom checker, iTriage, reports 50 million users each year. Symptom checkers ask a series of questions about your symptoms. Utilizing branching logic, Bayesian inference or other algorithms, they determine the probability of certain self-diagnoses to assist with triage. They are more or less capable of prompting patients with a potentially life-threatening problem, such as stroke or heart attack, to seek emergency care or reassure them that a medical visit is not necessary, for those with non-emergent problems, thereby saving you time and money. A study of 23 English language symptom checkers showed that only 34 percent of first diagnoses listed online, based on probability, happened to be correct, and were followed by the appropriate triage advice in only half of standardized patients.[41] Would you like to be in the 50 percent following the wrong advice, even for free? Probably not, so be aware of inconsistency and lack of reliability.

3. Check the credibility of your sources

Look at the website address (URL). The most reliable are .gov, .edu and .org:

- .gov identifies a US government agency, usually not supported by for-profit organizations, drug or insurance companies.

- .edu identifies an educational institution: a school, college or university.

- .org usually locates non-profit organizations (such as professional groups, scientific, medical or research societies, and advocacy groups).

- .com identifies commercial websites (such as businesses, individuals, pharmaceutical companies, and sometimes hospitals). Commercial sites can also offer accurate information but be careful about potential biases and secondary gains from advertising products or individual opinions, especially if websites are owned by companies offering health advice and selling products and services.[42]

If you are not sure about the website, look at the About and Contact us pages. What is the purpose of the website? Does it advertise certain products or services, ask you to schedule an appointment or buy products? Choose the information that comes from the organization that has expertise on the matter and doesn't solicit sales of services or products.

For example, I typed "weight-loss diet" into a Google search. It returned 1,440,000,000 results in 0.87 seconds.[43] The first four websites had "Ad" next to the URL and convenient phone numbers to call. I carefully avoided them knowing about the advertisement's purpose. The next were healthline.com, with bright pictures from the news, mayoclinic.org and hopkinsmedicine.org, followed by webmd.com and many others with a little Ad sign in front of the URL. As you might guess, I decided to stop on two websites: mayoclinic.org and hopkinsmedicine.org. Both are .org websites with the names of academic institutions I trust professionally.

I will tell you another secret to identify right away if the website has reliable facts.

In September 1995, some of the world's foremost experts on telemedicine gathered in Geneva, Switzerland, at the *Use of the Internet and World-Wide Web for Telematics in Healthcare* meeting to discuss how to deploy trustworthy health information online. A year later, the visionary experts created the Health On the Net Foundation (HON), a non-governmental organization, which, within two decades, has been solving two problems for the general public, medical professionals and web publishers: how to discern reliable health content and how to provide access to trustworthy information.[44]

Another goal of this organization is to establish its code of ethical conduct by giving, or not giving, websites supplying medical information HONcode certification, based on eight principles that are quite similar to the list of signs of reliability of health information that we just discussed, but HON does it for you. To be certified by HON, a website must formally apply for registration. If accepted, it must comply with all the principles enumerated in the HONcode. You can confirm that a site is registered by clicking on the HONcode seal, which should be linked to a registration status report on the HON site. By using a search engine in one of seven languages, on hon.ch/en, you will *only* generate websites with clear identification of authority, financial disclosures, cited sources, privacy information, and clear identification of advertisements. HON has been granted consultative status with the Economic and Social Council of the United Nations (ECOSOC).

You can use your usual search engines with the HONcode Toolbar extension seal (Google, Bing, etc.), which will be highlighted with red, white, and blue when you open a URL with trustworthy HON-certified information. If the website is not HON-certified, it would instead continue to be gray.[45] HONselect, another free Health On the Net Foundation tool, combines five information types—MeSH®, scientific articles, medical news, websites, and multimedia—into a single tool of focused and accelerated medical information searches. From my search on "weight-loss diet," only two websites came as HON-certified: mayoclinic.com and webmd.com.

4. Check who wrote the information and when

People prefer to hear directly from experts who have analyzed facts without "cherry picking." Does the published article name the author? Does the author or reviewer work for the institution that leads scientific studies or treatments of this condition or medication? What are this person's connections to sponsoring institutions and financial disclosures? Choose articles written by healthcare practitioners with expertise in the area. Don't be seduced by personal stories that may have a lot in common with your symptoms. It's just a story and isn't a reliable source. There are excellent websites dedicated to specific diseases owned by medical associations. Check when information was written—is it up to date? Are the studies cited in the article recent?

Health websites can be phenomenally misleading. Misleading can be harmless ("Epsom salts relieve inflammation") to potentially dangerous (recommending the use of supplements without knowledge of interactions with your other medications). Stay away from websites that promote their services and sell products under the skillfully created umbrella of educating about disease and treatments, using patient stories as examples of cures or names of authorities without evidence from well-supported, randomized controlled trials, and quality scientific information and citations.

5. Focus on evidence-based engines

These websites give the health information without advertisements. The National Library of Medicine, for example, is the world's largest biomedical library of health information for medical professionals, educators and, specifically, the public, since its founding in 1836. It has two free HON-certified services for the public: PubMed® and MedlinePlus. PubMed® contains (in most cases) brief summaries of articles from scientific and medical journals. For guidance from the National Center for Complementary and Integrative Health (NCCIH) on using PubMed, see How To Find Information About Complementary Health Approaches on PubMed. MedlinePlus collects authoritative information from the National Institutes of Health and other government agencies and health-related organizations. The Cochrane Library might be too detailed for the general public, but if you are looking for expert and evidence-based reviews and clinical trials, you'll find it in the Cochrane Database of Systematic Reviews (CDSR).

Google Scholar is a part of Google. It covers more than PubMed and includes books, articles, academic publishers, professional societies, and other websites. You might find full-text articles that are searchable. Click on Advanced search and type in your keyword. Under Settings, limit it to specific domains, such as .edu, .gov or .org, rather than .com to avoid commercial sites and improve the quality of the information you retrieve. To locate a full text, click on the link PDF, if available. By default, Google Scholar sorts by most cited and relevance.

Under Article, type "systematic review." This will give you a summary of all relevant studies over a health-related topic. You might see the words *systematic review*, *Cochrane review* and *meta-analysis*. Systematic reviews adhere to a strict design based on reproducible methods. They provide reliable estimates about the effects of interventions.

Cochrane reviews are systematic reviews undertaken by members of the Cochrane Collaboration, which is an international not-for-profit organization that helps people make well-informed decisions about healthcare.

Meta-analysis is the statistical analysis of a large collection of analysis and results from individual studies, and which you might find a little complicated. It usually helps to estimate the effect of treatment or risk factor.

When you choose either of those reviews, make sure they are recent. Choose one search engine and get familiar with it to be able to use it at the time of need.

CHECK YOUR HEALTHCARE INVENTORY:

1. Download the HONcode Toolbar to check the reliability of the websites that you use for healthcare information.

2. Bookmark the ones you find useful and reliable for future browsing, for example:

   a. nlm.nih.gov
   b. scholar.google.com
   c. medlineplus.gov
   d. familydoctor.org
   e. nccih.nih.gov/health

CHAPTER 6

DECEPTION OF SELF-DIAGNOSIS

Rose Cook loved Fridays; there were no worries about getting up early the next morning. This Friday she had a blind date and was being careful with her makeup. She thought she would never play the dating game again after 20 years of marriage. "Not too much, not too little, just right," she said, looking critically at herself in the mirror. It had taken her almost five years to recover from the betrayal of infidelity by her husband, her high-school sweetheart, whom she'd planned to spend her life with. *Jeans might be too tight.* Her attention turned to a touch of discomfort low in her abdomen. "Oh, no!" She felt a little urge to go to the bathroom. The urges didn't stop. She ran to the bathroom and when she sat on the toilet, she saw her urine becoming pink and eventually a little drop of blood came out.

"I have a urinary tract infection! Antibiotics usually take care of it. Could you please send the antibiotic to my pharmacy?" Rose asked the doctor-on-call. She seemed confident in the assessment of her symptoms and the treatments that had been successful in the past. She'd had the same symptoms many times. Less than two months ago, Rose had again typed in the Google search: "urinary frequency, urgency and low abdominal pain." The same answer came up: "urinary tract infection." Rose didn't have time to go to the clinic for the urine test, as the doctor-on-call recommended. "Why? The symptoms are typical," she replied. She'd had the same episode at least three or four times within the last two years. They always resolved after she'd taken antibiotics for a few days. She canceled the date and instead spent the evening taking trips to the toilet and having a hot bath, which seemed to make the urges better.

People tend to diagnose themselves based on their knowledge, past experiences, and information they find on the internet. More than one-third of adults in the US regularly use the internet to self-diagnose their symptoms.[46] It's hard to avoid the urge to find out the cause of symptoms when sources of health information are widely available with the accompanying "how to" and "DIY" advice.

Learning how your body works and looking for an explanation of your symptoms is a reasonable inquiry of knowledge. The inquiry usually starts with typing our questions into one of the typical search engines, but how reliable is this search? To answer this question, Mayo Clinic researchers searched Google, Yahoo!, and Bing databases to find information about eight of the most common acute conditions that patients presented with to urgent care clinics: chest pain, shortness of breath, abdominal pain, headache, fever, diarrhea, nausea and vomiting, and fainting. They identified 120 sites—15 for each symptom—and some of them, such as for chest pain, shortness of breath, abdominal pain, fever and fainting, gave potentially dangerous and life-threatening information. Every third site failed to identify symptoms critical for the diagnosis. No site contained a complete set of critical symptom indicators. Most importantly, there were no specific recommendations for further actions in almost half (42 percent) of the websites. When they were present, they were not rapidly identifiable and accessible and often lacked prescriptive guidance.[47]

Would I discourage my patients from looking up health information online? Absolutely not! I would caution, though, to not "name the disease" and make major health-related decisions based just on an internet search. Unsubstantiated information may lead to misdiagnosis, wrongful interventions, and delay of necessary treatments.[48]

Rose eventually came into the clinic after one of our doctors refused to follow her directions and insisted on checking the urine test first. The urine test confirmed the presence of blood even after the symptoms had resolved. As for the doctor-on-call, existing guidelines do recommend starting empirical treatment immediately for patients with uncomplicated urinary tract infections complaining of typical symptoms, without performing a urine culture test. In a cost-utility analysis, giving antibiotics seemed to be more cost effective than when a treatment decision was made after performing tests. It was thus concluded that a urine culture test may not be necessary based on its cost-effectiveness.[49]

The caveat was in the repetition of Rose's symptoms and her risk factors. Rose had a few "typical" symptoms of uncomplicated urinary tract infections: urinary frequency, low abdominal pain. She'd also had blood in the urine on and off within the last 12 months. After reading about the urinary tract infection on the internet, Rose concluded that if antibiotics reduced her symptoms, her "diagnosis" was correct. Her erroneous conclusion rejected other potential reasons for her symptoms. She was a smoker with a 20-pack per year smoking history and had stopped smoking two years ago. Her symptoms were persistent not because of recurrent infection, but because of bladder cancer, which she was diagnosed with by a urologist who performed cystoscopy (endoscopic study of the bladder) and bladder biopsy.

According to experts, we make most of our decisions using our unconscious mind. To survive the challenges of human existence through evolution, our minds have developed unconscious biases that influence our behaviors, or blind spots. When we make decisions about our health, we miss the truth by continuing to see life through the narrow window of those blind spots. Mo Gawdat, who isn't a psychologist or physician but an engineer, entrepreneur, and the former chief business officer for Google X, wrote the book *Solve for Happy*, which came out after the tragic death of his beloved son from a medical error. Using his engineer's logic and modern problem-solving skills, Gawdat described seven blind spots: filters, assumptions, predictions, memories, labels, emotions, and exaggerations.[50]

FILTERS

Our brain filters out redundant or impertinent sensory stimuli to prevent information overload, and this is controlled by the prefrontal cortex. It simply shuts down unwanted background and distracting noises from the environmental stimuli reaching the brain. Subtle symptoms of illness, such as being more tired than usual, a change in appetite, and fatigue, might get blocked by other worries (internal distractors), such as pressure from overwhelming work, taking care of others or financial burdens (external distractors). We don't recognize them until illness shows symptoms that are impossible to miss. We can break this blind spot by intentionally inspecting our own sensations and comparing them with our normalcy patterns to identify those that keep coming back.

ASSUMPTIONS

As an evolutionary survival skill, our brains have learned to cope by focusing on negative experiences to survive. We have learned to assume the worst to prepare us for defense. We view our assumptions as facts when they might be far from the truth or just partially true. "Something is wrong; it's probably cancer." We struggle when imagining the challenges of postoperative recovery when we're offered surgery. We assume that more tests are better and justify money spent for needless scans. We think that doctors don't care when, in reality, they haven't been notified about the results of the tests, or they don't know about our hospitalization, while the healthcare system simply cannot provide seamless communication of patients' related information to their doctors. Being aware of the true facts instead of assuming the worst would spare us from false expectations, expensive treatments, and the delay of medical care.

PREDICTIONS

Too often we refuse flu shots because "every time I have a flu shot, I get the flu." Is this true? You probably had light cold symptoms and didn't even go to the doctor's office to get a flu test. We convince ourselves that we need to take multivitamins daily to stay healthy instead of eating a healthy diet. Is that true? There is no data to prove it. We predict that if we eat five or six meals a day, we'll miraculously lose weight. Is that true? If you eat six meals a day without even experiencing feeling hungry, you actually consume a lot more calories and gain weight. Too often, our predictions are wrong and lead to undesirable actions.

"I have a green-color discharge from my nose after a few days of cold. I need antibiotics." Wrong! A sinus infection can cause clear mucus, and a common cold can turn it green. Cold is caused by viruses and almost always clears up on its own without serious complications. Antibiotics are not only ineffective, but often cause side effects. Get reliable information instead of believing common myths.

MEMORIES

"My father had diabetes and took insulin, and then he died. I might die too if I take insulin." Is it true that there is a connection between insulin and death? We might think it happened, but it's not a true story. Most likely, your father died from the complications of diabetes, which progressed to the end stages and affected his vital organs.

"I have the same pain in my low abdomen as I had during my last bladder infection," we say when we call the doctor's office asking for antibiotics. Is the pain really the same? Is it coming from the same body part in the lower abdomen? Pain signals trouble, but there are other organs in the lower abdomen besides the bladder that could also hurt. By believing in partial facts, we might reject much-needed investigation and get the wrong treatment.

LABELS

We label symptoms (headache, diarrhea or knee pain) with a wrong diagnosis (migraine, food poisoning or arthritis) and get misguided treatment. That happened to Rose for six months, delaying the diagnosis of bladder cancer. We quickly label experiences (fall, food, cold weather) as a reason to justify symptoms and avoid a visit to the doctor as an overprotective mechanism, without checking all the facts.

EMOTIONS

We are frequently guided by emotions instead of logic, such as by rushing into expensive and time-consuming emergency departments for symptoms of ear pain or worsening back pain instead of seeing a doctor the next day. We are afraid of shots, and yet they might prevent us from having painful and sometimes devastating infections. Is pain from a needle as bad as illness itself, especially if it can be transmitted to loved ones and make them sick? Once emotions, such as fear, attach themselves to decisions, they can become difficult to detach.

EXAGGERATIONS

To reduce surprise or avoid distractions from goal-oriented activity, our brains have learned to decrease the seriousness of unpleasant or unfamiliar reactions and increase the gravity of comforting ones.

Our cognitive appraisal system gets sidetracked under the pretense of a safer environment and fits our preconceived notions of reality. We tend to overestimate positive experiences, magnifying the truth and underestimating negatives. We conceal symptoms from clinicians, underrating the disease, just because we only have a few minutes for the visit, or we aren't ready to face the bad news. We count on weight-loss medication that will help us lose 30lb at once, overestimating the power of the drugs and downplaying more difficult-to-maintain lifestyle changes, such as moderate eating and increased activity. We exaggerate the opinions of certain doctors without questioning and stopping to seek other solutions, limiting our options for treatment.

Is it wrong to look up a potential diagnosis based on your own symptoms? Right or wrong, eight in ten internet users look online for health information including explanations of symptoms and available treatments,[51] driven by a genuine curiosity and desire to solve their own or family members' medical dilemmas. When you search for answers online, be aware of these blind spots. Bring up detailed information about your symptoms to your clinician, especially when those symptoms persist. Let the clinician make the diagnosis.

CHECK YOUR HEALTHCARE INVENTORY:

1. Gather the facts from your internet search about your symptoms.

2. Don't draw conclusions. Instead, prepare questions and talk to your clinician.

3. When you have done this, analyze your blind spots: filters, assumptions, predictions, memories, labels, emotions, and exaggerations. Which one(s) are yours?

CHAPTER 7

DECEIVING PERCEPTIONS

The perception of symptoms can play a more important role in our decisions than we realize. The beliefs we grow up with, or the perceptions we have acquired, might not be true or based on science but are powerful enough to make us act on them. Their familiarity makes them trustworthy. I grew up in Siberia where people lived nine months of the year in cold temperatures and were used to preserving their "inner heat," accustomed to cold temperatures being a *threat*. "Drinking icy water might cause a sore throat." "Don't turn on the air-conditioning, you could get a cold or flu."

Health perceptions define how we perceive our health. A recent diagnosis of hypertension and high cholesterol may elicit fear of complications of the illness, such as stroke and heart attack. This fear diminishes our feeling of wellbeing, and we feel more ill and more eager to stop health-affecting habits. We become compliant with medications, stop smoking, make efforts to lose weight and we exercise. Once chronic illnesses are under control, however, our health perception changes for the better, and we miss scheduled follow-up visits, stop medications, and return to habits that caused the illness in the first place. Perceptions are tricky; they can exaggerate or underestimate the reality.[52]

Carlos and Rita always came together to our Family Medicine Center. Both in their late-30s, they had grown up in Puerto Rico and moved to the US as teens with their parents. They didn't have children, but by the way Rita looked and cared about Carlos, I could see her nurturing instincts. Carlos looked like a "big" boy: stocky, but athletic, with dark unruly hair, long shorts that he wore even during cool seasons, a buttoned-down shirt, a tight belt with a cowboy buckle and hiking boots. He was an avid bicyclist who spent his free time exploring nearby mountains on his Stumpjumper trail bike, which he liked to brag about to our residents.

Carlos had a long history of diabetes, elevated blood pressure and cholesterol, but had learned to control them with medications, diet, and his weekly 30-mile bike rides. His visits to the office were short. On this occasion, his diabetes was well controlled, and his cholesterol and blood pressure were on target. His bright smile at the end of the visit articulated his pride in his sacrifices of regularly taking medications, following a good diet, and investing time in strenuous exercise. Rita didn't speak much during the visits but smiled broadly too, proud of Carlos for overcoming his health challenges. At the end of the follow-up visit, Rita gently touched her husband's elbow and said, "Tell her about you 'pooping too much'."

"Stop it! I started to eat a lot of fiber to get rid of the extra weight. You give me all those vegetables to eat, no wonder!" Carlos seemed embarrassed to talk about his stooling and cut the visit short.

During her own annual physical the following month, Rita asked "How many times a day is it normal to have bowel movements?"

"It varies," I answered. "A change in consistency of stool pattern or pain with bowel movements can be concerning, especially if there is weight loss, blood in the stool or any other symptoms. If you still worry about your husband, ask him to stop by and we'll figure it out."

Three weeks later, Rita and Carlos were back in the office. Carlos looked visibly uncomfortable and kept looking at his wife, who held his hand when he talked about his bowel movements, which had been increasing in frequency to five to six times a day, but were otherwise the same in terms of amount, consistency, color, and lack of discomfort. He didn't feel pain or fatigue, and his weight remained stable. "Carlos was adopted as a baby, so we don't know his family history," Rita said. She had already searched Google for "risk of colon cancer" and ended up thinking about symptoms of irritable bowel syndrome, a chronic illness of unknown cause, which shows up as diarrhea, constipation or both, and feelings of belly discomfort, cramps, gas, and bloating that improve after bowel movements. It was suggested in the same article that symptoms would improve if Carlos avoided a high-fiber diet. Rita had stopped cooking vegetables, and Carlos went back to his favorite meat and chicken. "Doctor, he just poops a lot, but no diarrhea or anything."

Carlos' physical exam was completely normal. We ordered the bloodwork to check for potential blood loss, and a highly sensitive fecal immunochemical test (FIT); a stool test that can detect even a small amount of blood. All tests, including his liver function tests and even inflammatory markers, came back as normal. He felt relieved when he received a call back with clear results, and he promised to see a gastroenterologist anyway, as I recommended.

Two months later, Carlos developed severe pain in the right side of his abdomen and blood in the stool. A large colorectal mass was found on the abdominal CT scan, performed in the emergency department. Only after that finding did Carlos have a colonoscopy that confirmed the suspicion of colon cancer. It was close to 12 months since Carlos had started experiencing frequent stools, which he'd ignored as not serious. He paid attention to his health, took his medications religiously, followed a diet and had an active lifestyle. He checked his blood glucose and never missed his visits. Carlos was focused on his known diabetes, high blood pressure and cholesterol. He'd found his own explanation for his frequent bowel movements, so didn't even talk to his wife for the first three or four months about his symptoms.

Carlos and I were dismayed at the colon cancer diagnosis. Why hadn't I made this diagnosis earlier? This is a question doctors painfully ask themselves many times throughout their years of practice. Human reasoning is prone to cognitive illusions, errors or, rather, irrationality. Perception-dependent reasoning allows us to align conscious attributes toward the desired vision of our health. The presence of chronic illness influences our health perceptions by focusing on certain symptoms and ignoring others.

Carlos noticed frequent stooling right away. His perception was that it wasn't dangerous because "this isn't diarrhea or constipation." In fact, he decided, "It might be a good thing because it'll help me to lose weight."

RISK PERCEPTIONS

People are frequently averse to unknown health conditions and new risks.[53] This may lead them to focus their attention on known and recognizable symptoms and fail to deal with less familiar symptoms.

According to psychosocial theories, there are three types of risk perceptions that predict motivation for actions and behavior change. If you perceive that your risk for cancer is low, you are less likely to agree to go through colonoscopy to prove it. Most people base the risk of health threats on some reason-based judgment that is invoked in health behavior, called *deliberate* risk. *Affective* risk perception refers to the feelings associated with the threat that we express as worry, anxiety or fear. "How fearful are you of getting these conditions in the future?" The presence of chronic illness influences our health perceptions by focusing on certain symptoms and ignoring others. When you struggle with elevated blood pressure, diabetes, or arthritis, you foresee complications from those diseases and think less about the risk of cancer, for example. Research shows that patients with chronic medical conditions are less likely to undergo cancer screenings.[54]

The third type is *experiential* risk—the perception of a gut-level feeling of vulnerability to a threat. "How vulnerable do you feel to the threat?"[55] From all three risk perceptions, *affective risk perception* is the strongest predictor of protective motivation, especially when deliberative risk perception is high as well. When we persistently worry about the threat of heart disease and are aware that our parents died from heart attacks, we are more likely to pursue lifestyle changes. But we also tend to ignore other issues that we are not focused on. "You can't see the forest for the trees!" Step back, look at the whole picture of your health with known and potential risks, based on your age, gender, place of residence, stress level and not only the illness you are already dealing with.

WHY KNOWLEDGE IS NOT ENOUGH

It's easy to feel lost, even when you've found reliable information on the internet, which adds more anxiety to already existing symptoms. It's also common for people to misinterpret and hyperbolize their symptoms and convince themselves that they have life-threatening illnesses.

Searching for health information may indeed cause distress and add more uncertainty about your doubted condition. For those who are already distressed and anxious about their health, excess medical information may be taken the wrong way. Driven by fear, some people turn to excessive searches for comfort about their health issues, instead of turning to a health professional.[56] This is particularly true of patients who are convinced that there is something dreadfully wrong and who have put a considerable investment into being "sick." When people seek reassurance about their health and instead experience the misleading and confusing effects of unreliable websites, they get into a cycle in which repeated online searches increase distress and anxiety.

Convinced about misleading diagnosis or treatment, some may begin to search for medical practitioners who will share those beliefs and ask to order expensive tests to confirm their viewpoint. If doctors don't agree, they continue "doctor shopping," or may turn away from conventional to alternative medicine, which may also delay treatment and cause a progression in illness. But there have also been times in my practice when patients were right, suspecting certain illnesses and finding the right treatment, despite other professional opinions. I have made faulty assumptions, cognitive errors and have learned to listen and trust my patients' judgments. Diagnosis is a clinical puzzle, which patients and doctors have to put together without discarding the pieces but making sense out of them. The patients' role is to bring the "puzzle pieces" to doctors and fill in the gaps of clinical analysis by pressing for answers.

Andrew was a freshman at the College of Charleston, a liberal college of the arts with a reputation as being a party city. With uncombed jet-black hair and a shy smile, he reminded me of a bird, trapped in the wilderness.

Andrew grew up in a family with two loving parents and a little sister in the suburbs of Virginia. His mother left her teaching job as soon as his sister was born and devoted herself to her family. She dutifully took her kids to pediatricians, never missing scheduled exams or immunizations. Andrew remembered his family dinners involving discussions about the day's ups and downs, and laughs, which always gave him a feeling of belonging to a family that protected, supported and cared. His grit, good health and athletic skills paid off well in the form of scholarships, which he excitedly accepted.

In the clinic, Andrew didn't make eye contact with me, and seemed nervous. "My stomach hurts right below my rib cage. I read about GERD on the internet and tried Tums. They helped for a while. Last month the pain was on and off, now it hurts every day."

"Have you lost weight?"

"I lost a few pounds."

"What do you eat for dinner?"

"I love pizza. I eat burgers, French fries. Salads don't keep me full. I snack on chips. I don't like soups. I drink a lot of coffee to stay awake."

Andrew's heartrate was racing in the early 100s, blood pressure was borderline 135/90. He looked tired. The sclera of his eyes was tinted slightly yellow. His palms were moist, and his fingers trembled during the handshake. His abdomen was slightly tender.

"What do you think is happening to you?" I asked, trying to dig deeper to confirm my inner feeling that Andrew wasn't talking about the many other problems that lay beneath the stomach pain.

"Probably ate something wrong in the cafeteria. I read on the internet that stomach pain can be an ulcer. I do drink beer, just a few with friends, more on weekends. I went to see a psychiatrist, who found that I have ADHD and put me on Ritalin. I didn't have ADHD when I was in school, it just started my first year in college. My grades could be better, if I could focus … I had to retake two courses last summer."

"Exercise?"

"I don't have time. I lost my sports scholarship. I have a problem going to sleep. It's hard to get up in the morning, so I missed a few morning classes."

My suspicion of depression and anxiety was confirmed by high scores on standard instrument testing. People usually fail to admit the real amount of alcohol they consume. A "few beers" in the social history brought to light serious alcohol problems when we used the validated questionnaire. His elevated liver enzymes revealed signs of inflammation of the liver, triggered by alcohol. Alcohol and caffeine contributed to his anxiety and depression, his elevated heartrate and blood pressure. Ritalin, which was prescribed to improve his focus, mixed with alcohol, not only boosted the effects of anxiety and impaired his sleep, but also impacted his cardiovascular system by raising his heartrate and blood pressure. Instead of improving, his focus and learning abilities worsened, leading to degrading school performance.

Like every student, Andrew was skillful in searching the internet for health information. But his true health problems of depression, anxiety, and alcohol use weren't even included in his search.

WHY DO WE HAVE DIFFICULTY MAKING THE RIGHT DECISIONS WHEN WE POSSESS THE KNOWLEDGE?

The Institute of Medicine has declared that nearly half of American adults may have difficulties in "acting on health information,"[57] calling it the "health literacy epidemic."[58] Health literacy is not just the ability to find information, but to understand it and use it for health-related decisions.[59] Even when you find necessary information on the internet, you have to be able to understand unfamiliar medical terms, interpret risk evaluations, and figure out the diagnoses and available treatments.

Andrew had high literacy skills but struggled with his low health literacy. People with high literacy skills, but who have recently immigrated to the US, may still not be able to respond adequately to their health concerns and have a low health literacy. Some would rather tolerate symptoms than show a lack of knowledge. Twenty-six years ago, like many immigrants, and in spite of my medical degree, I found myself confused about every step of US healthcare, from making an appointment to picking up prescriptions from the pharmacy.

Robert Hamm, PhD, spent decades studying how doctors make rational decisions about their patients, and how patients make rational decisions about their health. In his studies, he showed that "patients lack both the facts about the uncertainty of particular diseases and especially the skill of revising their own estimates of those facts to produce an updated estimate of disease probability. Patients without this understanding may make mistakes, such as worrying excessively about a low probability of disease or assuming they are free of a disease that has not yet been ruled out."[60]

For example, let's say you identified the problem "I have hair loss." You search for hair loss causes and treatments on reliable websites, and you realize that there are different types of hair loss. "I don't have patchy hair loss, or male pattern baldness, as described in some sources, I have thinned hair." The action step—What can I do about it?[61]—starts with adapting knowledge to your particular dilemma: "What treatments are available for my hair?" Then, you acknowledge and assess the barriers to knowledge use: "Changing my shampoo and conditioner to a sulfate-free one will be more costly and might not solve the problem." The barriers might stop you right there before any action steps are made. Or you can assess potential harm or get professional medical help.

Clinicians could provide you with reliable facts that you understand, as well as with solutions on how to bypass the barriers. If projected harm is minimal (changing the shampoo), you use trial and error and learn from your mistakes ("I will stop using braiding to reduce tension and will wash my hair once a week instead of every other day"), monitor the outcomes and finally continue applying this "knowledge to action" framework to other health questions. If you determine that risk of trial is harmful or time is limited, seek professional medical help. The most effective decisions about health are collaborative, based on patients' experiences, physicians' expertise, and mutual trust.

Making a clinical diagnosis is like solving a puzzle: you must have all the pieces. Patients bring the symptoms, doctors add the exam, their knowledge of illnesses, and medical decision-making skills to fit all the pieces together and make a true picture of "illness."

CHECK YOUR HEALTHCARE INVENTORY:

1. What do you think your level of health literacy is?

2. Test your health literacy level with the Agency for Healthcare Research and Quality's simple tool (see General Resources). The Rapid Estimate of Adult Literacy in Medicine—Short Form (REALM-SF) is a 7-item word recognition test to quickly assess health literacy and compare with your assumptions.

PART TWO

YOU AND THE DOCTOR

"The doctor of the future will be oneself."

ALBERT SCHWEITZER

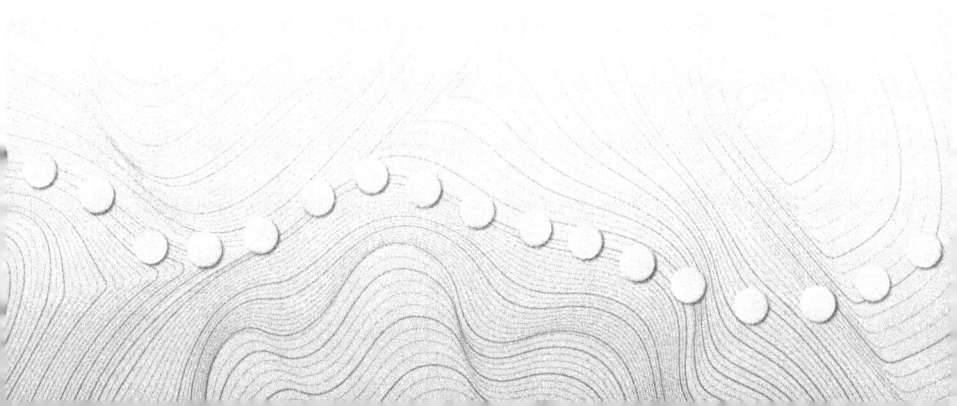

CHAPTER 8

TELL YOUR STORY

The first time I heard about Gloria was on a Friday afternoon. Residents and clinic staff were getting ready to leave for the long Fourth of July weekend. The weather promised to get better, and we were talking about the beach, sun, and fireworks, although I could still hear the thunder that made the windows shake. Rain was pouring down in the parking lot. "Look," said Amanda, my nurse, who'd worked in the University Family Medicine Center since the day it opened its doors to the community. Amanda knew every patient, remembered every former resident or even attendings who'd left, retired, or died. She loved good stories, and her memory did not fail to keep them. I looked at the window, covered with rain. The rushing wind crossed the opening door of a black Cadillac and almost bent the large umbrella that the bold man with broad shoulders in the trench coat was holding in front of the passenger seat.

Then, a leg and the four-inch heel of a Manolo Blahnik pump appeared. Both feet touched the puddle of water, covering pointed toes. "This is Gloria," announced Amanda, when we saw the woman in a hat and long white trench coat step out of the car. She looked like a model who had just come from the catwalk somewhere in Milan. I didn't know what to make of Amanda's announcement, containing tones of both admiration and warning. I rushed to the computer and pulled up my next patient's medical history. Gloria Rosewell, 44 years old, married, college graduate, former smoker, no children. There was an endless list of medical problems from fatigue, nausea, back, joint and chest pain, to shortness of breath. This seemed the most comprehensive list of all kinds of complaints a human could have.

Amanda, who had a talent for making people share the details of their lives, updated me on the Rosewells' "social history." Bob Rosewell was a prominent NYC banker, who one day unexpectedly retired and left NYC to live on a farm that belonged to his parents at Wadmalaw Island, with beautiful river views and close to Kiawah Island's park beaches. Even after moving to South Carolina, Gloria never stopped being a New Yorker, with her fashionable pumps, dresses, and scarves, looking different from the easygoing and laid-back southerners.

Since that rainy day I treated Gloria for fibromyalgia, fatigue, joint pain, migraines, nausea, constipation, shortness of breath, allergies, elevated blood pressure and palpitations. I referred her for consultations to a cardiologist, a gastroenterologist, a pulmonologist, a rheumatologist, a neurologist, and an allergy specialist. Every time she had returned angry, because "nothing worked" and she "felt miserable" while looking at me with her sad, dark, deep-brown eyes, almost as if she was trying to transmit the message that I perpetually failed to understand.

One day, Amanda gave me her warning look for trouble, and said, "Gloria is asking to talk to you."

"Put her in the schedule for today," I responded, knowing that the phone conversations we'd had didn't let me see Gloria's nonverbal communication, which had so far provided me with more guidance than her words.

When I walked into the room, Gloria was alone. Her dark curly hair was down, which made her almost unrecognizable from the skillfully constructed hairdos she usually wore. She did not have her typical high-heeled shoes or fancy dresses on. In her white button-down, jeans and dark flats she looked like a teenage girl. She still did not make eye contact. Her eyes were attached to her hands, which she squeezed together so tightly that her intertwined fingers started looking dark.

"I grew up very poor, in a big family in Farmerville, Louisiana. My dad and my brothers worked on the farm. I always dreamed of getting out of the small town and living in a big city. I studied hard, played basketball, and got a scholarship to study at the University of Louisiana in Lafayette." She was speaking fast, as if she was scared to be interrupted and wouldn't be able to tell her story. *Wow!* I was thinking, *Gloria is from the South.*

"Yes, I am from the Deep South," she said, as if reading my mind, "and I used to love it." She took a deep breath. "I was gang raped. The first day I arrived at Lafayette." Then she looked at me with those dark eyes full of tears and pain. "I've told no one. My husband doesn't know. I had to have an abortion and couldn't have children after that. I moved to New York, far away from the South, and worked as a waitress in a restaurant until I met my husband." She stopped talking and a shadow of a smile brightened her face. "He thought that moving back to the South would make me happy."

Doctors are accustomed to listening to patients' stories. I find patients' stories the most rewarding experience of my job. Fortunately, they also provide the biggest clues to diagnosis of the ongoing illness and treatments that may work. But what to do when this amount of grief comes out? Grief that has been hidden and buried at the bottom of someone's soul for decades. Now, I could explain the myriad nonspecific complaints of pain at different places, episodes of palpitations and chest discomfort, followed by normal tests that were run by multiple specialists and myself. Gloria denied physical or sexual abuse every time she was asked, and I still don't know why she confessed that day, but now the mask was off.

"I've done hundreds of tests and procedures to discover illnesses in my body. I've visited doctors who couldn't find anything wrong. I know what's wrong with me. I am angry. I am sad. I have been carrying the burden of pain and injustice too long. I am mad with myself that I wasted so much time looking outside when I knew from the beginning what help I needed. The statute of limitations has expired. Can you help me?" We cried and made a plan.

Gloria talked to her husband, and he became her biggest coach and companion in her healthy initiatives, from jogging to meditation and yoga classes. With the help of a psychologist and cognitive behavior therapy, Gloria's outlook on life changed. She founded a girls club in her local church and opened a boutique where her sense of fashion found many happy customers. She faithfully continued a small dose of antidepressants for two years. The medical complaints, one by one, cleared up like clouds from the sky, proving well-known wisdom that your story is the most powerful and cost-effective diagnostic tool available.[62]

"The medical history brings enough accurate information to make a diagnosis in about 75% of patient encounters even before performing a physical examination and additional tests," wrote Nobel Prize winner, Dr. Bernard Lown, in his book, *The Lost Art of Healing*.[63] It also doesn't cost thousands of dollars, like PET scans and MRIs do. Your story, with facts leading to symptoms, is the information that only you possess. If you don't share it with your clinicians, they might lead you to the wrong path, just as Gloria went to multiple specialists and underwent myriads tests, which took years of her life. Gloria did not disclose an important part of her history for two reasons: she felt pain and the shame of being raped, and she did not connect it to her somatic symptoms for a long time. When doctors have a patient who does not provide a truthful history, this itself becomes the biggest challenge and creates a huge potential for errors.

There are other obstacles in the healthcare process that make patients' history invisible to physicians, who're desperately looking for the clues to diagnoses.

Remember how your medical history is collected when you visit a doctor? You answer the questions in the paperwork given to you by each individual office. Dentists ask more detailed questions about your teeth, ophthalmologists about your eyes, dermatologists about your skin … hoping that primary care doctors can put all of this together. You don't write about the factors that precipitated certain symptoms, thinking you may share it later. Medical staff review your answers, interpret it into medical language and put it into medical records for doctors to verify during the visit. Most people don't realize that snippets of history that have been provided to different physicians don't get dropped automatically into one big computer, accessible to all medical professionals. These pieces of information cannot be pulled up by other physicians unless all your life you have been visiting one health system with the same medical records, which is almost impossible.

Unfortunately, electronic medical records (EMR) don't yet talk to each other. Errors can occur at every level of entering, organizing, and saving your health information. As a result, many facts that could help with diagnosis and treatment can be missed, misinterpreted, entered inaccurately or saved at the wrong place in the medical records, where they might not be easily identified.

Yes, technology is not perfect, but it's also not the major reason why patients' stories are not being heard by clinicians. In two recent national surveys of 4,510 Americans, 60–80 percent admitted they hadn't been forthcoming with doctors about information related to their health.[64] Some people are unsure what to say and what not to say when asked about their medical problems, often providing incorrect information, such as, "I don't have high blood pressure or high cholesterol; they're controlled by medications," and therefore they avoid listing elevated blood pressure or cholesterol as an existing medical condition. Some are not ready to face medical issues, hoping that if we don't talk about them, they will not exist.

Scott Warren, who was tall with a touch of gray hair, in his early 60s and tanned from regular time at the golf course, came into the clinic dressed impeccably in his jeans and black cashmere sweater, the sleeves rolled up, showing one of those expensive watches men measure each other by. Scott was a pure impression of confidence and success. He'd grown up in Michigan, and his parents owned a tracking company. Scott and his three brothers were assigned chores and duties related to the family business, no matter what school or other obligations they had. He learned work ethics and an attitude for hard work, encompassed by, "I can do it." This had helped Scott get to Wharton School of Business, then get an internship at Goldman Sachs and eventually start his own hedge fund. Scott was fortunate in his corporate job and retired in his 50s. He moved to the South Carolina suburbs and settled in a comfortable ranch away from the noise of NYC.

Scott's story sounded like one of James Bond's adventures to me. He owned gun auctions, rode Harleys, raced sailboats and flew his own airplane. There was also a pretty woman in the picture: his lovely Serbian wife, who traveled with him all over Europe. He was overweight, and I could sense the tickling smell of an expensive cigar.

"I'm in perfect shape, Doc. My wife, she's a nurse, sent me to establish care, just in case," he started. Scott was scheduled for the annual wellness exam. He filled out the office intake forms with "past medical history" given the brief answer "no" in all sections: no chronic medical problems, no complaints, no surgeries, no to smoking, no to alcohol, no family history of heart disease or cancer. "I feel great. I play golf three times a week. I have my Scotch now and then and stopped smoking ten years ago. Well, I do smoke cigars with the boys on occasions. I eat well. My parents never had heart issues and lived till their late 80s. Life is good, Doc."

"Your blood pressure is up, 165/90." I glanced at him, triggering an irritated response.

"It's always up in the doctor's office, but normal at home."

Talking about a patient's weight can be a delicate problem. Tackling it during the first visit might push patients away as a "negative" message. I noticed Scott's BMI of 34 and waist circumference of 45 inches (normal is below 40 inches for men), which alone can be a sign of increased risk for heart disease and diabetes. From his sneer, I gathered that comments about weight loss would not be met with enthusiasm and decided to wait till the next visit after the lab results were back. I handed Scott a summary of the visit with a suggestion to monitor blood pressure for two weeks, follow a DASH (dietary approaches to stop hypertension) diet,[65] as well as tips on how to stop smoking and lose weight.

A few days later, I called Scott about his laboratory results. His blood glucose was slightly elevated, and cholesterol was on the high side. Together with uncontrolled blood pressure, his risk score for atherosclerotic cardiovascular disease was high.[66] "We could decrease the risk to 'low' if we treat your elevated blood pressure, cholesterol and work on the diet," I suggested.

"I'll fix it," Scott said. He missed his next follow-up visit. Four months later, I received a phone call from an inpatient resident. At the end of 18 holes of golf, Scott had felt "indigestion." It didn't resolve after he popped a "purple pill" of omeprazole. "I had it from time to time for almost a year," he later told me. In 20 minutes, Scott had collapsed. 911 was called. Scott was rushed to the hospital where he was diagnosed with myocardial infarction.

Could I have prevented his heart attack from happening? I felt defeated and guilty. Why didn't he tell me about the chest pain he had from time to time?

The sun was shining through the window when I walked into his hospital room on the fifth floor. "I'm sorry, Doc," were his first words.

Scott's cardiac catheterization showed complete blockage of the left anterior descending artery (LAD), the largest coronary artery. It runs almost half of the blood carried by all heart circulation. Atherosclerosis or clots that blocked this major vessel had caused serious damage to large areas of the heart muscle. Myocardial infarction in LAD is sometimes called a "widow-maker." His cardiologist placed a percutaneous stent to restore the blood flow in that powerful artery and another smaller artery. To reduce risk of clogging of the stents, Scott had to take a blood thinner and medications to control his blood pressure and cholesterol.

"I've always been in control of my life. My father was never sick, except once after falling off his horse in his 70s. He taught me to be 'strong' physically, work hard and do what I love. I thought I could handle it. Yes, my blood pressure was off on quite a few occasions. I tried to take fish oil capsules because my cholesterol was off the last couple of years. But they gave me heartburn. I didn't tell you about any of those. Sorry, Doc."

As with many "wanna be perceived as tough" men, Scott didn't want to complain about trivial symptoms, such as lingering chest discomfort, confusing it with indigestion. He hoped he'd found the solution in a self-prescribed "purple pill." Through his entire life he had succeeded in overcoming risks through toughness and perseverance. People frequently close their eyes on the human body's vulnerability under the pressure of age, genetics, and self-destructive habits. Scott was in the driver's seat of his health like he drove his cars, boats and planes—taking risks. He did not tell his story because it did not fit the narrative of himself in his mind.

CHECK YOUR HEALTHCARE INVENTORY:

1. Ask yourself if you are keeping any "secrets" from your clinicians that could be helpful for them to understand you and treat you more effectively.

2. Clinicians need your "true story," not for judgment but for clues for diagnosis, so be ready to provide it.

CHAPTER 9

COMMUNICATION DANCE

A conversation with a patient:

"What brought you here today?"

"I want to make sure I'm okay."

"Are you feeling well?"

"I think so."

"Do you have pain anywhere?"

"Yes, I have a headache. I'm so tired. I also fell last night. My knee swelled."

I would compare patient-doctor conversations with a dance. In the above conversation, a stoic patient gives a vague answer to the question "Are you feeling well?" The physician takes the lead and responds with a more specific question. "Do you have pain anywhere?" This opens the gate to a flood of symptoms.

Patient-doctor communication is not just any dance, but a tango, full of emotional twists, unexpected turns and pauses. The dance tells a story and conveys emotions. Dancers communicate in meaningful ways, creating connections. Depending on the relationship between the patient, illness, and doctor, it can be an indifferent or emotional conversation. "It is the medical dialog that provides the

fundamental vehicle through which the paradigmatic battle of prospective is waged and the therapeutic relationship is defined," wrote
Debra Roter, Professor of Health Policy and Management at Johns
Hopkins University, who spent most of her professional life studying
patient-doctor relationships.[67] In her studies she showed that based
on how a doctor asks questions and responds to patients' emotions,
patient activation and engagement will happen, making the patient
feel free to speak and participate in a dialogue and reveal the clues
necessary for the doctor to make a clinical diagnosis. If the patient
is cut off prematurely or constrained, however, then the doctor may
miss something important.

Gloria and I had had many dialogs, but only when we touched
her emotional side strongly enough, and she felt our emotional connection was safe enough, did she tell me her story. It would be foolish
to deny that emotions are present at every level of the patient-doctor
encounter. The emotional layers in medicine, however, are far more
nuanced and pervasive than we may like to believe. In fact, they can
often be the dominant layers in medical decision-making, handily
overshadowing evidence-based medicine, clinical algorithms, quality control measures, even medical experience. And "this can occur
without anyone's conscious awareness," wrote Dr. Danielle Ofri in her
book, *What Doctors Feel: How Emotions Affect the Practice of Medicine.*

We don't always get to "chase" and "tell" about the problem we
want the physician to help solve. Even if the clinician asks the right
questions, the patient may be not feeling *safe* enough to tell their
story because of their emotional state. Only when a physician understands the patient's emotions will the story be told.

The dialogue between a patient and a doctor also occurs on nonverbal levels: whether the patient likes the doctor and whether the
doctor appears to like the patient. It comes from the physician's facial
expressions, common gestures, whether they are kind and welcoming
or formal.[68] We expect clinicians to take a lead in asking questions.

Clinicians are trained to actively gather a patient's chief complaint and past medical history by following the pattern of "what, where, when, how much, and what it's associated with or caused by..." Do you have pain? Your great toe hurts? When did it hurt? Did it hurt before? Two years ago? Did you fall? No? Etc.

Almost automatically, clinicians match patients' complaints with their mental library of potential diseases with similar symptoms, then return to the patient to clarify the details. This helps to build a potential list of diagnoses with similar symptoms, called differential diagnoses. It might be followed by a "twist and turn" in the right direction if empathetic communication between a patient and a doctor happens. If the physician doesn't ask and we don't tell, important facts will be hidden from the physician's radar. If the physician doesn't express enough empathy, we might not feel heard and will not provide information necessary for the correct diagnosis, sending the physician to the chase of seeking the confirmation of the wrong hypothesis in myriad expensive tests. As a result, diagnosis might be delayed or missed, and costs trumped up. When patients come in with an already gathered medical history and list of medical concerns, it not only paves the path to the diagnosis but also saves time and money from unnecessary testing, spares you from anguish about non-existing risks and gives you more time with your doctor for issues that matter.

Patient-doctor communication is frequently called a *therapeutic relationship* because it has the power to influence treatment and healing. It may fail, as any treatment, or succeed. Relationships between the doctor and a patient are mutually chosen. Like a dance, you can both step in one direction or another. Even paternalistic relationships, where you feel unequal to the doctor, can be shaped and negotiated to a more active relationship. Instead of telling your doctor, "Yes, I will do that," let your doctor know that the plan of treatment does not agree with you and why. This will prompt your doctor to think about alternatives.

A consumerist model of the relationship, with the power resting with the buyer (patient), which limits the physician's role contingent on patient preferences, also has little chance of succeeding, unless a balance between the roles is achieved. The most functional model of the patient-doctor relationship is described as medically functional, informative, facilitative, responsive, and participatory.[69] Patients want expert information from doctors in an understandable, useful, and motivating manner that will help them cope with overwhelming uncertainty that comes with an illness. We expect exchange of information, which relates to the building of a partnership, where the physician facilitates and welcomes the patient's active participation. Similar to when partners are moving in the same direction, motivated by the same music on the dancefloor.

EFFECTIVE COMMUNICATION

So, why are some communications with a doctor less efficient and effective at problem-solving than others? Thinking about a potentially threatening illness doesn't make us good communicators. While nervous, we may forget about symptoms and questions we'd planned to talk about. There are two other barriers in the way when telling your story and getting medical care: the first is the time allocated for your visit; the second is the number of people involved in your care, called "transitions."

A medical assistant meets you first, obtains your history and documents this in the medical records. Doctors may not communicate with medical assistants between seeing patients. If you haven't told your complaint or question to the medical assistant accurately, or they didn't write about it in the EMR, or they placed the information in the section the doctor doesn't look at, the clinician will not know about your concerns or details, which makes a big difference for the diagnosis. Being prepared to repeat all the details at every level of questioning is a reality that we cannot avoid in most practices.

Primary care patients' appointments are usually scheduled for 30 minutes for new patients and 15 or 20 minutes for established patients, depending on the type of practice. Specialists' appointments are usually longer. Only one-third of the allotted time is actually spent by the doctors asking and answering questions and examining patients. The rest (10–20 minutes) is spent on documentation in EMRs and clerical work.[70]

Researchers from Texas A&M Health Science Center and Harvard Medical School used an innovative videotape analysis to estimate that the primary care office visit lasted around 15 minutes, with the longest being in the academic medical center (23 minutes) and the shortest at the solo practice (9.7 minutes). During the visits, patients and doctors spoke *slightly more than five minutes* each on average, covering about six topics. Patients in the solo practice spoke on average for less than two minutes.[71] Speed dating would be a similar experience when you express concise personal information in a little longer than one minute.

Time is a barrier not just for patients. Clinicians feel the pressure of time even more. While listening to you, clinicians translate your symptoms into medical vignettes, create a list of potential diagnoses that the symptoms would fit, called differential diagnoses, then ask more questions to focus on the most reasonable diagnosis, and make a plan for treatment. They also document all of this in the EMR. They also write orders, referrals, and prescriptions, which must be ready before patients leave the office. This is a pretty long to-do list. Expert physicians, because of continuous reflection, have a much shorter path to the right diagnosis by using relatively few pieces of clinical data.[72]

There is another obstacle in the way of your concerns coming out and where relevant clinical information can be missed—clinicians are active communicators! They are skilled in asking closed-ended questions and redirecting patients' initial description of concerns. Studies on patient-doctor communication showed that in only one out of 51 visits did the patients have the opportunity to complete the opening statement in the process of physicians collecting the patients' description of concerns.[73] Physicians redirected the patients' opening statement after a mean of 23.1 seconds. Once the discussion became focused on a specific concern, the likelihood of returning to complete the agenda was very low (8 percent). As a result, patients may miss the opportunity to present relevant facts of their story and physicians miss out on gathering important patient data.[74,75]

When we are nervous or feel uncomfortable, or are distracted by pain, we forget relevant facts. That's why it's always good to have your major facts written down: medical problems you have been diagnosed with, surgeries, medications, allergies, and family history and symptoms you want to address. Sometimes a trusted friend can help fill the gaps and ask pertinent questions.

Time constraints add further pressure on both physicians and patients, creating more barriers for communication between a doctor and a patient. Analysis of videotaped visits has shown that during a little over 15-minute visit, the physician and patient talk for an equal amount of time; five minutes each. The longer patients talk, the more uncertain physicians feel about the diagnosis and the plan of treatment. Patients who require more time for their medical history end up receiving less time than they needed for an explanation of the plan of treatment.[76]

Nonverbal communication, or old-fashioned "bedside manners," also matter. While completing tasks of documentation, ordering tests, and sending prescriptions, all within a short period, physicians might not keep eye contact, and we might misinterpret that as "the doctor doesn't listen or doesn't care." That might not be the right impression, but if we feel mistrust, we might not be convinced enough to take the medication or agree to a procedure that would improve our health outcomes.[77] Don't make conclusions too quickly; see if the impression stands over time. Ask the physician to clarify the plan for you. Let them know what you are interested in and find out what orders are being placed and tests ordered.

KNOW WHAT YOU WANT

Communicating your wishes is especially important when we get older. A quarter of all medical spending occurs in the last year of life.[78] Worse, higher spending in the last week of life has been associated with a poorer quality of death,[79] while many interventions may be conflicting with patients' preferences.[80] According to researchers from the University of South California, patient choices are frequently based on physicians' attitudes to treatments and not necessarily on their own preferences.[81] Patient willingness to withdraw life support appears to be related to physicians' attitudes about end-of-life planning.[82] If patients don't want to or have not discussed their preferences with their doctors, they will most likely end up suffering from unwanted, aggressive care.[83]

So, how do doctors make their own decisions about end of life? They get sick and die, the same as anyone else, with one difference in that they know what is going to happen during illness, especially terminal.[84] Doctors are familiar with side effects of chemotherapy and cutting-edge technology of lifelines, tubes, monitors, and advanced equipment that will keep your body in a vegetative state indefinitely.

When facing their own death, doctors mostly don't want to prolong life if it cannot be lived fully. They also have a clear understanding of their health conditions and what they may encounter in the future, where laypeople might have false hopes and beliefs. This clarity and personal experience make their own decision-making simpler. They have options to try all available treatments, but they usually choose the minimum: comfort from pain and being with family. Families frequently want "everything" to be done for their loved ones, without clearly understanding how unreasonable that "everything" can be for someone who will experience it. How much pain and discomfort from resuscitation, feeding tubes and medications will their loved one experience before their eventual death happens anyway, days or weeks later.

In the fee-for-service medicine model, excessive treatment on the principle of "do everything" can generate a large bill for the family to pay after the death of a loved one. Doctors are fully aware of this and are realistic about making choices around the type of end-of-life treatment for themselves. Doctors usually know what they want and communicate it clearly.

My surgeon mother was only 44 when she was diagnosed with metastatic breast cancer. In the era of no mammograms in Siberia, her cancer was diagnosed late, when metastasis had spread into the bones. I couldn't understand at the age of 19 when my mother refused to eat five days before her death. Chewing caused her excruciating pain in her jaw, ravaged by metastasis. "I will also stop eating if you don't eat," I told my mother, knowing that she would never want me to be hurt. She started eating soft food after two days, seeing her only child starving. I wanted to prolong my mother's life. She did not. She knew that brain metastasis would take the best of what she possessed: her mind. Dr. Gallo, from Johns Hopkins University, studied doctors' wishes about life-sustaining treatments and said, "Surgeons wanted the least interventions, internists and pathologists were in the middle, and psychiatrists wanted the most."[85]

"No chemo, only radiation to take care of pain, and no pain meds," my mother said to her medical team. "I want my mind and my looks with me until I die."

Accustomed to helping patients with decisions about death, doctors usually have no problems making their own decisions, more likely refusing unnecessary treatments with a preference for minimal care. They communicate their wishes clearly by leaving orders with directions to be followed, informing their own doctors and family. Dr. Wittink, with colleagues from Johns Hopkins University, showed that physicians are more likely than the general public to create advance directives, living wills and laying out specific plans for care.[86]

My mother had chosen her favorite simple black dress and high-heeled shoes for the open-view casket with the same quick precision as she did her treatments. She wanted to portray the same confident look even in death, knowing that she would be viewed by her colleagues, students and patients in the university lecture hall. I was a first-year medical student and religiously followed her instructions, which distracted me from the thoughts of losing her. She succeeded in her intention of communicating her message clearly to me and her doctors: "Focus on what matters."

What can you do to avoid these obstacles and make communication with your physician effective? Establish a therapeutic relationship with your primary care physician. If you don't have a primary care doctor, find one (keep reading this book for advice). Your goal is to put your story forward and make sure it's delivered. Anticipate all the above barriers and prepare to communicate the facts as clearly as you possibly can. That's why writing a list of symptoms is helpful. Focus on what matters the most. Schedule another visit if necessary to discuss less relevant issues.

SHARING IS EMPOWERING

It can be frightening for some people to make big decisions about their health. "Share your pain," was taught to me by Dr. Kurlov, talking metaphorically about gathering opinions of colleagues about difficult clinical cases. Getting advice from your doctor as a partner is not only more satisfying, but also cost effective. Doctors bring medical knowledge and experience to the table. You contribute the knowledge of your personal goals, fears and struggles. Why is this treatment the best option for me? Why at this time? What are the alternatives? Conversations like these help to make the best medical decisions.

Jenny Turner had just turned 87. Dressed in her tennis skort, a t-shirt with the attractive logo "living life" on it, and a ponytail sticking out of her blue cap, she carried no extra weight and looked at least 20 years younger. Brisk movements of both hands during our conversation revealed an Italian communication style. She came to see me with her 65-year-old daughter and five-year-old great-granddaughter. By the smiles on their similar faces, I could feel the love they shared. I was the third primary care doctor they'd visited that week.

At 87, Jenny had not been seriously ill, but had colds and tennis injuries until six months ago, when chest pain made her go to the ER. She was not only diagnosed with myocardial infarction but was found to have a complete blockage in four major coronary arteries. After the open-heart surgery, she spent two weeks in bed, which was unfamiliar to her. Before the surgery, she was used to walking three miles every morning and swimming in the pool for at least 30 minutes a day for six months of the year. She helped to raise her grandchildren and their children, sang in the church choir and cooked dinner for her daughter's family every day.

After the surgery, she developed back pain that was spreading to her leg like an electric shock, making sitting unbearable. She felt dizzy after taking medication, which was prescribed by the surgeon for the pain. She tried heat and ice. An x-ray showed shortened vertebrae and signs of osteoporosis. A radiologist suspected a compression fracture in the lumbar spine and recommended an MRI to clarify the reasons for the pain. The word fracture terrified her, but not as much as the perspective of any surgical interventions. "I don't care if I have a fracture. I don't even want to know."

"What do you want to try to achieve? What is most important to you?" I asked bluntly.

"I don't want to do anything now, just try to improve my pain and functioning. I don't want pain pills that would make me dizzy or sleepy." Jenny didn't want to know a "correct" diagnosis either. At least not now. We decided to try topical anti-inflammatory ointment. She found a physical therapist who patiently worked on stretching her back muscles and strengthening her core. She agreed to see an acupuncturist, whose techniques took the edge off her pain. She returned to the choir in the church, which brought moments of happiness. We agreed that, if pain persisted at an excruciating level, she would call me. She did not call. A year later, I received a call from her daughter. Jenny had had a good year, returned to all her activities but tennis, and she managed to learn golf. She had died in her sleep.

When decisions about testing or treatments have to be made, physicians let patients know about the available options with the associated pros and cons related to the patient's medical condition. Instead of silently agreeing with the physician's offered option, you should ask questions. Why is this option the best for me? What is going to happen if I wait or choose another option?

I have seen many patients who trusted the opinions of less-experienced clinicians and agreed with offered treatments, dismissing therapies offered by attendings with years of experience. Sometimes it's the same culture, language or even age or gender that the doctor and patient have in common, which generates a trust that makes shared medical decisions effortless for both parties. The clinician and a patient share a personal connection with each other. Patients might express feelings and information about self, goals, and values. The physician explores the patient's values and beliefs and recognizes the importance of the patient's ability to understand. Both discuss information about the risks and values of the medical service, then they share control and negotiate the decision. After the decision has been made, implementing health decisions resides with patients.[87]

When a doctor acknowledges trust in a patient, the patient feels responsible for the outcomes. The patient's empowerment brings more value to the treatment, making it more successful. It's not always an easy process, and it may take time to reach a decision that will be supported by the physician and the patient. Frequently, it's a doctor's communication skills, knowledge of the patient and the established trust between them that play a role in the success of shared decisions, rather than a doctor's expertise and extensive knowledge.

CHECK YOUR HEALTHCARE INVENTORY:

1. Clearly communicate the reasons for your visit, not only to the staff, but to the doctor.

2. If there are many reasons, prioritize them.

3. Be prepared to focus on the most important issues and schedule another visit for the rest.

4. If specific questions need to be answered, gather all available medical facts in a summarized form.

CHAPTER 10

CONFESSIONS

Melinda Homer was an engineer who came to our clinic complaining of tingling and numbness in her right hand that had been getting worse. It was her dominant hand, and she was quite anxious about the symptoms increasing over the last few months. She had tested negative for carpal tunnel syndrome, which was suspected, but was still being treated for it by wearing a wrist brace, though without any improvement. She had neck MRI imaging done, suspecting nerve damage in her cervical spine. It found age-related degenerative changes and was followed by a recommendation of two six-week courses of physical therapy, which made no impact on her symptoms. When she started having numbness and tingling in the other hand, her worry escalated, and she requested a full workup for multiple sclerosis.

Dr. Cao was a third-year resident, known for her detailed approach, her patients' lengthy visits and being late in the clinic. Melinda became frustrated when Dr. Cao kept asking questions instead of simply giving her the referral for a brain MRI, which she expected.

"Do you remember when and how the symptoms started?" Dr. Cao asked. Melinda confirmed an absence of trauma and doing her usual activities at work and at home. "Did you lose or gain weight?" Dr. Gao kept asking. "Oh, yes. My husband and I became vegetarians

two years ago after his heart attack, and we eat mostly whole foods."
Vegetarians are at risk of vitamin B12 deficiency if they don't supplement this or eat fortified breakfast cereals, soya milks, soya/veggie
burgers and vegetable margarines. Vitamin B12 is required for the
function of the central nervous system, healthy red blood cells and
DNA synthesis.[88] Too little vitamin B12 can lead to anemia, with
symptoms of low energy and tingling and numbness in different parts
of the body.[89] Melinda's initial blood test did not show anemia and
her vitamin B12 level was not checked. A repeated blood test confirmed that Melinda's vitamin B12 blood level was two times the minimal level of normal, and methylmalonic acid, a functional marker
for vitamin B12 deficiency, was highly elevated. After four weeks of
vitamin B12 injections, Melinda's tingling and numbness were gone.

We usually don't comment on our habits during visits unless we
are asked about them. Having knowledge of someone's dietary habits
can give clues to diagnosis and risk factors for heart diseases, migraine
headaches, asthma, allergies, neurological and many gastrointestinal
problems. Some of us simply don't want to acknowledge the problem or risks, especially if they are related to smoking, alcohol intake,
recreational drugs, traumatic experiences or sexually transmitted illnesses. We withhold the truth, despite understanding that the information we provide is indispensable for making a diagnosis. In two
national surveys of 4,510 US adults, every second patient misrep-
resented their dietary habits, alcohol intake and physical activity.[90]
Approximately one in ten smokers and 5.8 percent of former smokers have withheld their smoking status from their clinicians.[91]

Disclosing our habits might seem like an invasion of privacy and
an invitation to be judged. There is also the perception of the social
undesirability of certain habits, like smoking, and the fear of health
insurance penalties from disclosure. Some don't disclose their habits
for reasons of embarrassment, they don't want to hear how harmful
the behavior is, don't want the clinician to think they are a difficult

patient or take up more of the clinician's time.[92] Twelve percent of patients withheld information from their physicians for information security concerns.[93]

How is this information useful for your future? If you are a smoker, even formerly, clinicians can calculate your health risks based on your pack per year smoking history by multiplying the number of years you have smoked by the amount of packs per day of cigarettes. A high pack-years number correlates with a higher risk of cancers, heart disease, stroke, diabetes, chronic obstructive pulmonary disease, osteoporosis, peripheral vascular disease—and premature death. Smoking causes nine out of ten lung cancer deaths.[94] Screening for lung cancer is easily available now from the age of 50. If you have a more than 20-pack-a-year smoking history, and currently smoke or have quit within the last 15 years, physicians would start annual lung cancer screening with low-dose computed tomography (LDCT) and identify lung cancer at an early stage, before symptoms occur.

Alcohol consumption is a leading cause of preventable deaths in the United States[95] and can impact a variety of diseases, from cerebrovascular to depression, anxiety, and gastrointestinal disorders. Excessive alcohol use was responsible for more than 380 deaths per day in the US each year during 2015–2019. But even brief interventions in the primary care setting have shown a net reduction in alcohol consumption of 12–34 percent.[96]

Some 48.2 million people, or about 18 percent of Americans, used recreational drugs at least once in 2019.[97] Close to two-thirds of marijuana users in one study initiated medical cannabis by themselves to treat their anxiety, depression or insomnia instead of asking physicians for help.[98] Patients frequently substitute cannabis for prescription drugs, often without their clinician's knowledge, delaying diagnosis and appropriate treatment. In the surveys of those who use marijuana for medical purposes, only every third patient informed their doctor.[99]

Why should doctors know about marijuana use? Cannabis is a drug that interacts with multiple medications (for example, warfarin, valproic acid, benzodiazepines, theophylline). It might interfere with the treatment of your atrial fibrillation, asthma, bipolar disorders, and seizures. Doctors may prescribe you a medication that might not work or give you dangerous side effects, just because it interferes with cannabis. It may increase risk of bleeding in patients taking warfarin, cause liver injury while taking with valproate for seizures or bipolar disorder or cause breathing difficulty due to the decreasing effect of theophylline in patients with asthma, emphysema or chronic bronchitis.

When treating ADHD, a physician may start increasing the patient's dose of stimulant, which would increase the risk of insomnia, anxiety, and palpitations, instead of advising to decrease marijuana use. I see many young people in the office seeking treatment for poor focus and attention deficit to improve work productivity and memory, asking to be prescribed stimulants. Many use cannabis at the same time. Marijuana, by directly affecting the brain, can jeopardize memory, learning, attention, decision-making, coordination, emotion, and reaction time.[100]

The reasons for withholding health information that could help physicians make the right diagnosis are simple: we don't want to be judged or seem difficult, and we want to make the best impression. Close to half the people in one study lied about their diets, exercise habits, sex lives or adherence to treatments, mainly out of embarrassment.[101] We know that and teach young doctors to "double their patients' reports about alcohol use and halve the reported amount of exercise" for a more accurate picture. Almost two-thirds of people withhold information about the use of complementary medicine methods and the supplements they take, worrying about physician disapproval.[102] Patients with worse health and chronic medical conditions are more likely to withhold information.[103]

Would you withhold information about the issues with your car when you take it to the mechanic to get fixed? Probably not. Confess! Tell your physician about your past and current habitual behaviors: diet or lack of it, emotional eating, binging or sedentary lifestyle. Calculate your pack-per-year smoking history and ask about your risks and what can be done about it. Make sure cannabis is on your medication list in the electronic medical records, which automatically checks for interactions. Marijuana is a chemical that interferes with many medications and may reduce or increase their effects, making them potentially dangerous.

Even though it might feel uncomfortable to tell all about recreational drug use, you need to confess. There might be solutions for medical problems hidden behind your habits and risks that you are not aware of. Physicians don't judge; they need to know about your risks to use them as cues for the correct diagnosis.

CHECK YOUR HEALTHCARE INVENTORY:

1. Write down a list of your former and current habitual behaviors (diet, exercise, activities (min/week), smoking (pack/day), recreational drug use (name/frequency, last used), unprotected sex, others, and share with your doctor.

2. Discuss the impact of your habits on your health and medical problems with your physician.

CHAPTER 11

CALL OUT THE RED FLAGS

Symptoms are signals of new sensations, individual subjective experiences, which only you can feel. They are different from the already familiar feelings of "being well," or our status of normalcy that we are accustomed to. Only you can recognize the symptoms' quality and location or notice that they are coming back and with how much intensity.

Symptoms cannot be seen and do not show up on medical tests. If you don't bring them up with details when communicating with your clinician, the early signs of the illness might not be recognized.

Clinicians "spot" certain symptoms from your story that fit into the list of potential differential diagnoses (possible conditions). The more details of symptoms a patient describes, the more certainty will be added to the diagnosis. Clinicians scan patients' symptoms by systems and call it a "review of systems." They start with general symptoms (fatigue, fevers, weight loss), then move to respiratory (everything about your breathing, such as congestion, cough, wheezing, difficulty of breathing), cardiovascular (chest pain, palpitations), neural (headaches, dizziness, numbness) and gastrointestinal (stomach pain, diarrhea, nausea), going systematically through all the systems.

Don't let the doctor guess—do your part in recognizing symptoms and their details: severity, location, pattern, associations and what makes them better or worse. For example, a headache can be sharp, dull, stabbing or pulsating. It might be associated with nausea, increased sensitivity to light or sound. Only you can notice if the headache starts during physical activity. While primary exercise headaches are usually harmless, secondary exercise headaches can be caused by bleeding or tumor in the brain. Just this little detail might prompt your clinician to order an MRI scan and identify it, while most of the time headaches do not require brain imaging at all.

Symptoms can be acute if they start and progress quickly, such as pain in the ankle after a fall, or vomiting. Try to focus on those that keep coming back. Watch for patterns and try to come up with a description instead of labeling with a diagnosis you found online. Symptoms are like bricks of cues that build up your history of illness. Doctors call it the "history of present illness" (HPI). That history has a power of 60–80 percent for making the right diagnosis.[104]

When you recognize the symptoms of illness, the next question is, "Are they dangerous?" Doctors separate symptoms from *signs of illness*. When symptoms of illness can actually be observed by you or others, they are called signs. Signs can be seen (redness, swelling, bruising, shaking, droopy face), heard (wheezing, voice change, confused speech, snoring), smelled (breath or wound smell) and felt (tenderness to touch, sound produced by tapping, clicking when moving the joint, feeling heat during the touch, elevated temperature). It might be a lack of a familiar sensation—vision, hearing, touch, movement.

Signs of illness are similar to the signs on a highway. You might miss them if you're busy thinking of something else. You have to be vigilant and paying attention. *Red flags* traditionally mean signs of impending danger. Red flags in medicine are signs of serious or even life-threatening illness and call for urgent action.

For the last two days, Kyle Grant had felt nauseous. The pain in his stomach was annoying. It didn't allow him to focus on his new marketing plan that he had to discuss tomorrow with his team. At 31 years old, slim and athletic, Kyle had never been sick except for one or two colds a year. "No more nachos again, even for business reasons!" he was telling himself, blaming his recent business dinner for his persistent nausea. Kyle put on a sweater despite the temperature in the office of 75 degrees. The pain in his belly became sharp. *What is going on?* He wondered. He typed "nausea, abdominal pain" in a Google search, and "when should I be concerned?" which produced a long checklist. Reading this took his worries away. "I don't have black, tarry stools or vomiting, chest pain, neck pain or shoulder pain. I have no bloody diarrhea either. Great!" Kyle decided to give his gut a "rest" by not eating anything and just drinking water. He tried to prod his stomach in different places; it was slightly tender everywhere, but more below his belly button than above.

Kyle called his primary care doctor's office. "Most likely food poisoning," concluded the triage nurse, recognizing the impact of his "social dinner with tacos and nachos." Her voice was reassuring: "Drink more water, avoid fatty foods and take it easy. Call if symptoms don't resolve in a couple of days or worsen." She also promised to talk to the doctor. Doctor Young called back in a few hours. Kyle liked his doctor. He was about his age, athletic, enthusiastic, and approachable. Dr. Young was also interested in wellness. They had even shared their exercise routines during Kyle's last annual physical.

Dr. Young also went through his checklist: "You have no chronic medical problems, according to your medical history. You didn't vomit; your appetite was good. You had normal bowel movements and no fever, and no blood in the stool." The doctor's voice was optimistic. "Most likely this is a 'stomach flu'. I've been seeing it a lot lately. Drink more water and advance your diet slowly," finished Dr. Young, adding, "Kyle, don't hesitate to go to the ER if symptoms worsen, or any of those worrisome signs we just discussed occur." Kyle was asked to call back if the symptoms lasted longer than two to three more days. The doctor's confidence took care of Kyle's worries, but not the symptoms.

The next day, Kyle couldn't concentrate on any of his secretary's questions. "You don't look right," said Cary, Kyle's middle-aged, quiet secretary with a concerned look on her face. Kyle had hired her as a favor to his friend. She clearly didn't fit into his high-paced and full of energy office. Cary was older than everyone, had three teenage daughters and her dress style reminded Kyle of his mother. Whether it was the fact that usually "silent" Cary made a comment, or the sign of "trouble" in her eyes that reminded him of his mother, or maybe her concerns matched his worries about the increasing pain, but Kyle decided to go to the ER.

The ER was busy during rush hour, so Kyle felt relieved when the nurse informed him that his "vital signs, temperature, blood pressure and pulse are great, so hopefully you'll be out of here soon."

"Another abdominal pain case," warned the nurse, a few minutes before Dr. Ryan Murphy was about to sign out at the end of his shift. The ER rotation was Ryan Murphy's last transitional year rotation. He was scheduled to start his dream radiology residency next week.

Dr. Murphy checked the electronic medical records. There was no information about this new patient, just today's vital signs. He liked to get the medical history from the previous records before seeing a patient to anticipate potential diagnosis. It could save so much time! Unfortunately, this time he had to start from scratch: history and physical exam. He thought about the game of soccer he was supposed to join with his team in an hour at the recreation center.

Dr. Murphy was tired, and, from his unshaven face, he knew it was obvious that he looked like he'd been there for a while. *Looking a little pale, dark circles under the eyes*, he noticed as he shook Kyle's hand in greeting. *Abdominal pain, nausea after eating out, no fever, no diarrhea, no vomiting, healthy guy*, went through his mind while listening to Kyle's story. The abdominal exam was brief but more painful for the patient than he'd anticipated as Kyle almost jumped when Dr. Murphy's hand came off his belly abruptly.

"Rigid abdominal wall, but the pain isn't localized in the right lower side of the abdomen. Hopefully, laboratory tests will reveal more information," he reported to his upper-level resident while placing the orders at the computer station. When the orderly with a wheelchair asked Kyle to get in, Kyle assumed that the lab tests were abnormal, and a CT of the abdomen was the next step. Kyle was glad that the investigation was going quickly. Vomiting inconveniently started when Kyle reached the radiology suite, and he felt pain like a sharp knife around his belly button. Everything happened quickly after the CT scan.

"You need surgery, Kyle. It's acute appendicitis," said a surgeon, rushing him to the OR. Fifteen minutes later, Kyle was on the operating table, sending prayers to God and his good luck that made him go to the ER instead of waiting for "worsening of his symptoms."

Appendicitis is the most commonly seen abdominal emergency in the ER, requiring surgery.[105] The symptoms often overlap with other conditions, some of them self-limited, such as viral gastroenteritis, or stomach flu, making the diagnosis challenging.[106] Those medical conditions with similar symptoms of abdominal pain require watchful waiting with hydration as the only necessary measure. Some, such as urinary tract infections, can be treated conservatively as an outpatient with medications, and others may require surgery.

On Monday morning, when Dr. Young, Kyle's original PCP, found out about Kyle's complicated ruptured appendix, he felt guilty and distraught. "How could I miss acute appendicitis? I wouldn't have if I'd brought him to the clinic to be seen. I know Kyle, he's healthy and is a reasonable guy. I counted on his judgment. He didn't ask to be seen. There were no red flags."

WHAT ARE RED FLAGS AND
HOW DO YOU RECOGNIZE THEM?

"The Japanese railway system is considered as one of the safest in the world," wrote James Clear in his book, *Atomic Habits: An Easy & Proven Way to Build Good Habits & Break Bad Ones.* As each operator runs the train, they proceed through a ritual of pointing at different objects and calling out commands. This process, known as "pointing-and-calling," is a safety system designed to reduce errors by up to 85 percent and cuts accidents by 30 percent. The train operators must use their eyes, hands, mouth, and ears to notice problems before something goes wrong. The trick that the brain does to make pointing-and-calling so effective, is that it *raises the level of awareness of problems from an unconscious habit to a more conscious level.*

When some of your symptoms keep coming back, they whisper, "pay attention." You may try to push those little whispers away, but they are like a nagging voice telling you, "Hmm, something might be off. These headaches are new. I didn't have them last month and now I have them every other day," or "this pain in the flank keeps coming back." Ignoring the whispers, especially when they approach with stubborn persistence, is an invitation for trouble.

The term "red flag" is used figuratively as a warning of danger. Some signs of red flags are general: being pale and having severe pain, profusely sweating, passing out, difficulty breathing, having a seizure, profuse bleeding, and others. Some might be related to specific illnesses.[107] Abdominal pain, especially if not severe, is not always a red flag, but in combination with fever, vomiting or an inability to pass gas or stool, could be a sign of severe inflammation in the gut or a bowel obstruction.

What would a clinician be looking for if Kyle was seen in the office? The same things that Cary, Kyle's assistant in the office, and Dr. Murphy noticed in the ER. Sometimes we call it a "sick or toxic" look. A sick look can be present independent of the diagnosis: skin being pale—with a tint of blue, gray or yellow—damp skin, sharpened facial features—especially the nose—dry lips, sweat on the forehead, dark circles under the eyes, eyes closed, delayed reaction to the voice, troubled breathing—either shallow and fast, or deep and unsatisfying—frequent breaths that involve muscles of the face and neck, or that bring all of the chest up and down, weakness of muscles, altered speech.

Cary, Kyle's assistant, was attentive enough to recognize the missing pattern of normalcy in her young boss, and instead she saw his new sick look. From her experience in raising three children, she noticed he was looking pale, with dark circles under his eyes. She also noticed differences from his usual behavior patterns and interpreted them correctly: he was dressed in warm clothes despite the warm temperature in the office (chills and potential fever?), refusing to order lunch (nausea?), and a lack of focus (pain?). Mothers and wives learn to pick up on these patterns by watching their loved ones during daily routines and, thanks to them, tell their concerns to clinicians.

There is a pivotal point at which we decide whether our bodily changes might be signaling a serious health problem. Researchers named this period *"symptoms appraisal."* The presence of these signs should prompt us to act immediately by seeking a professional medical evaluation and immediate interventions. Unfortunately, our uncertainty about our judgment accounts for the majority of total delay of medical care. Even when patients notice symptoms that require medical attention, nearly one-third avoid seeking medical care. Depending on perception and our general tendency "to worry" or not, some of us minimize symptoms for a longer period of time, while others might exaggerate them.[108] In studies by Dr. Stephen L. Ristvedt and his colleagues from the Washington University in St. Louis,[109] a longer "symptoms appraisal" period was marginally associated with less education and a younger age. This makes sense as we often don't believe in health threats when we are young.

Jessica Roth was a typical teenager, 16 years old, busy in school and her swim team with training sessions almost every morning before classes. To avoid the inconvenience of monthly menstrual periods, she asked for oral hormonal contraceptives, which gave her 84 days of not having to worry about menstrual pain and bleeding. Two months later, after a training session, she noticed unusual dizziness with a slight headache on the right side. "Most likely, you have a migraine as I do," reassured her mom. Her coach sent Jessica to see her PCP. "Migraine," was also the conclusion of her physician. She was advised to take over-the-counter (OTC) Excedrin or Motrin and returned to the training sessions. After another session, she lost her eyesight for a few minutes. Her mother, familiar with her own migraine symptoms, thought that it might be an atypical migraine, which she had also read about on the internet. It was a morning when Jessica's mother was on her way to work and a long wait in the ER seemed an unwelcome solution for symptoms that had already resolved. She also dreaded keeping her healthy, athletic daughter at home.

Jessica was brought to the ER the next day with an inability to speak, right-sided weakness, and she was not able to walk. A cerebral angiography showed occlusion of the part of her internal carotid artery and both anterior cerebral arteries, as well as the left internal carotid artery, caused by a thrombus—blood clot.

This 16-year-old teenager had suffered a stroke, something we don't think of in young people. Investigations showed that Jessica had a revealed protein C deficiency, same as her aunt, who had died young. Protein C deficiency is a cause of thromboembolic disease, and the oral contraceptives had triggered the blood clot development. Arterial thrombosis is less common than venous thrombosis, and the symptoms had fooled her mother and her PCP, which prevented an ER visit when she had a transient ischemic attack (a warning sign of a future stroke) earlier.

ACTION APPRAISAL

Even when we identify red flag symptoms, we do not always rush to get help. Instead, we frequently bargain with ourselves instead of seeking care immediately. Researchers call it "action appraisal."[110] But why?

There are three main categories of reasons, according to Jennifer M. Taber, PhD, and researchers from the National Institutes of Health. First, we are swayed by general mistrust of doctors, unfavorable past experiences, and the "hassle" of healthcare, in addition to a fear of serious illness. Second, we don't want to believe that it's a serious illness, and third, we think our symptoms will improve over time. However, most of us frequently take medical risks because of a lack of resources, health insurance, money, and time.[111]

We bargain, looking for options that will save us time and money; for example, we send messages through the patient portal, hoping that a doctor will solve the problem. What may be an urgent issue for you, might get in line with all other routine messages about prescriptions, refills or referrals. Patient portals are not created to communicate symptoms, advice might come too late and would most likely be to see the doctor anyway. We call doctor-on-call. Discussing your clinical situation is always helpful for urgent cases, but a doctor-on-call doesn't know you well, may not have access to the details of your medical history and would rather make decisions with heightened risks to be safe, and will therefore send you to be evaluated in the ER. The general advice is to see *your* doctor, who knows you, works best. Identification of red flags point to danger; help to estimate the urgency of the situation and act on it by seeking the right help.

CHECK YOUR HEALTHCARE INVENTORY:

1. Do you have symptoms that have been lingering for a while?

2. Write them down, document the details: what, where, when, how much, and schedule a visit with your clinician to seek an explanation.

3. Are there any red flags? Call them out and act on them.

CHAPTER 12

THE DIAGNOSTIC JOURNEY

Waves crashed close to our white stucco house with the red window treatments. It seemed like the waves could pick up the house my mother and I stayed in, in Odessa, Crimea, and take it deep into the Black Sea. The thunder was loud, shaking the house. Bright-blue lightning was getting closer and closer. I was 15. The house was surrounded by vines, supported by posts and trellises heavy with ready-to-pick grapes. My mother was sitting in the dark leather chair across the window that I was staring at, mesmerized by the battle between the wind, water, and light. A bright, thin, sparkling-blue arrow came from the window toward my mother. Her body jerked, but she continued sitting with her head down. I have no memory of what happened after. I guess shock and fear took it away. "I survived the lightning," she later jokingly said about this experience.

The next day, the Black Sea was quiet and innocent, like the storm had never happened. I was stretching at the beach next to my mother when she told me, "You see this?" She was pointing at slightly bluish-red skin with a popping out vein on her leg, which seemed to be tender when she pushed at it. "This is called thrombophlebitis. It's pretty superficial, but this is my third one this month."

"Why do you have this?" I asked.

"I guess, something is going on in my body," answered my doctor mother, feeling comfortable with the uncertainty of her acknowledged symptoms. Later, in medical school, I learned that Trousseau's syndrome commonly indicates migratory superficial or deep thrombosis or blood clots traveling from one place to another associated with any malignant disease.[112] Three weeks later, my mother was diagnosed with late-stage breast cancer at the age of 44. The question that puzzled me for years was, why did she not diagnose her cancer earlier? She was a good doctor!

Uncertainty refers to a lack of definite knowledge, a lack of sureness. Both luck and risk are related to uncertainty. Luck is a *force* that brings either fortune or adversity. Thinking about luck, we acknowledge the role of chance in uncertainty, leaving us passive witnesses to potential outcomes.[113] The word luck rarely comes up during doctors' visits. We talk about risks to bring uncertainty under control by trying to prevent diseases, and by making diagnosis of illness early to avoid complications.

The reality is that luck plays a bigger role in our health than we would like to acknowledge. And, yes, we can't control it ... yet.

"Our health is subject to luck in four different ways," wrote American philosopher Thomas Nagel in his famous book, *Mortal questions*.[114] First is the phenomenon of *constitutional* luck—the kind of person you are, your genetic predisposition, your immune system, your personality and abilities you are born and raised with. Second, health is a subject of *circumstances*: pandemics, injuries, allergic reactions. The other two deal with the causes and effects of action: luck in how we are exposed to certain circumstances (secondary smoke, food poisoning, using preventive care), and luck in how we act on those circumstances in terms of unforeseeable consequences (poor surgical outcome, medication side effects, medical error).[115]

Uncertainty is a factor in diagnoses. The word *diagnosis* comes from Greek, meaning "a distinguishing, or a discerning, between two possibilities." Diagnosis is a process that patients and clinicians go through to identify the nature and cause of physical or mental discomfort of illness, by evaluating symptoms, signs and findings from the physical exam. If the diagnosis is still uncertain, physicians order diagnostic tests to bring more certainty to the cause of the symptoms.

The diagnostic journey starts with the clinician asking you a series of questions about your symptoms. The more details you contribute, the shorter and more cost-effective this journey may be. When your symptoms are acknowledged and detailed (what, where, when, how and how much), clinicians translate them in their minds into medical vignettes to compare with the similar vignettes in their personal "library of knowledge." If your complaint is "low abdominal pain," for example, after a series of questions your story gets translated into: *A 36-year-old female with a two-day history of low abdominal pain, urinary frequency and urgency without fever or back pain. List of potential diagnoses: urinary tract infection, kidney stones, sexually transmitted diseases, bladder cancer (less likely).*

The next step is to check your past medical history for certain illnesses and identify risk factors for them. After more questions, we add more certainty: *no history of kidney stones, no issues with kidneys in the past. Smoking for 15 years is a risk for bladder cancer, but unlikely at this age. Divorced, started dating and there was a new sexual partner three weeks ago. No hot flashes, no medications, but multivitamins.*

In Western medicine, the human body is divided into systems: neurological, respiratory, cardiovascular, endocrine, immunological, musculoskeletal, and others. As mentioned before, doctors review these systems in addition to the system that is most likely involved (in this case genitourinary) to determine what other parts of your body could be affected. Is there vaginal discharge? When was your last menstrual period? Could you be pregnant? Have you gained weight recently? Have your legs swelled? Was the sexual intercourse protected? In this case, if you answered "no" to all those questions, the list of potential diagnoses is still the same, but the probabilities of diagnoses have changed. Sexually transmitted disease becomes a front runner. Urinary tract infection? First time kidney stone? Maybe.

What will happen if you don't share the fact that you had unprotected intercourse with a new sexual partner with the clinician? Or if the clinician, who doesn't know you well, avoids uncomfortable, intimate questions about risk of STD because they are under a time pressure? Urinalysis performed in the office will not identify potential chlamydia or gonorrhea infection. STD screening tests for chlamydia and gonorrhea might not be ordered. Antibiotics, most likely prescribed for a bladder infection, will not cover chlamydia infection, and you will continue having symptoms, or potentially may develop complications and may transmit the infection to others.

The next step is to perform a physical exam, which provides important signs of illness. A thorough history and physical exam in almost 80 percent of cases can lead to the correct diagnosis, leaving only 20 percent for laboratory and imaging tests.[116,117]

In simple cases, clinicians don't need multiple tests to assure diagnostic certainty prior to initiating treatment, such as for a simple cold, nasal congestion, elevated blood pressure, skin infection, laceration or back pain. Adding laboratory or imaging tests helps to rule in or out other possibilities, but they are not always necessary or cost effective in every case. There are situations where diagnosis is close to 100 percent correct, such as with cancer, pregnancy or some infections. The gold standard is to examine a tissue, secretion or blood sample by laboratory testing. Tests are most likely necessary to determine the extent of the illness.

If suspicion for a certain diagnosis is strong, physicians might recommend starting treatment with a plan to then check on the feedback of the treatment to refine a working diagnosis.[118] If the treatment doesn't work as expected, physicians seek help from more tests and referrals to experts and other specialists.

Patients frequently wait for primary care doctors to refer them to a specialist without being aware of why their clinicians have referred them to a particular physician or medical practice. In an ideal world, the consultant should be chosen because they are the best qualified and are readily available to serve the patient. However, medicine is far from being ideal. In my experience, consultants' availability, clinical acumen, personal relationships, and habits are driving factors, with the ability to see a patient expeditiously being the most common.[119] There is an aggressive economic pressure from the health systems and insurance companies that the physicians are under. For hospital systems, employed doctors' referrals for specialists' consults, surgeries and imaging services are vital sources of revenue. Employed PCPs are frequently driven by "loyalty" pressure to keep business within a hospital system, even if an outside referral might benefit the patient more, could be done faster and for a better price.[120]

FINDING AN EXPERT

So, what should you do if you have a rare medical condition, or in spite of multiple doctors' visits, labs and tests, you have exhausted the options but feel that the correct diagnosis is still being missed? You might need to find an expert.

That's where a physician's experience and expertise come into play. "Experts see the world differently," wrote Joshua Foer in his highly acclaimed book, *Moonwalking with Einstein: The Art and Science of Remembering Everything*. "They notice things that non-experts don't see. They home in on information that matters most and have an almost automatic sense of what to do with it." My colleague Professor Clive Brock, from the Medical University of South Carolina, practiced medicine for close to 40 years, and rarely was he wrong in his diagnosis. His dark eyes looked almost through patients when he talked to them. "Pancreatic cancer," he concluded after a few minutes talking and examining our admitted heavy-built patient, whose sclera was slightly tinted yellow. "Why not just biliary stones?" asked one of the residents. "You will see." And, yes, we did. After laboratory tests and CAT scans, Dr. Brock's diagnosis was always correct.

It is acclaimed by Malcolm Gladwell, in his book *Outliers*, that there is a 10,000-hour rule of intensive practice to achieve expert level. I doubt that is correct for the medical field. After a quick calculation, 10,000 hours equates to little more than three years of practicing, if we assume physicians work nine-hour days. All physicians must achieve the highest level of competency in their field to make decisions about someone's life. They also have to adapt to medical ethics, "best practices," evidence-based science, as outlined in the clinical guidelines, and have the communication skills to make the right diagnosis, convey it to a patient and come up with a treatment plan that will be accepted and followed.

If you disagree with where you're referred, you still have an option to contact academic medical centers and "big name" institutions for consultation instead. Known for their research, large academic institutions, such as Emory University, Duke University, Mayo Clinic and Cleveland Clinic, provide consultations online upon patient and physicians' requests. For difficult diagnoses, there are innovative programs such as NIH's Undiagnosed Disease Network (UDN), and consultative programs at the Cleveland and Mayo clinics, which participate in national or international research and offer additional opportunities to discover entirely novel diseases.[121] Looking for an expert? Find one.

An example of this was Nico Kostopoulos, a successful real estate broker. When he learned he had fatty liver disease, he attributed it to eating too much lamb, which his Greek family indulged in every weekend. He didn't worry about it, until fatigue ate his usual energy away. It became hard for him to move around because of shortness of breath and leg swelling. His cirrhosis, or inflammation of the liver, progressed quickly, and soon he was dependent on blood transfusions to supplement blood he was losing from varices (dilated veins) in his esophagus.

Iron overload from frequent blood transfusions added more complications. Trips to the hospital became routine events. Helen, his wife of 20 years, always accompanied him, and relentlessly looked for other options, including a liver transplant. She refused to believe the hospital physicians who said that Nico wasn't a candidate yet, as she saw how his health was fading away. "My five children need their father. Nico is so weak, sometimes he doesn't recognize his children." Tears showed in her eyes. Toxins, not cleared by the cirrhosis-damaged liver, built up in his brain and caused Nico's mental confusion; a condition called hepatic encephalopathy.

One day, Helen took an unresponsive Nico to the hospital and was told, again, that his model for end-stage liver disease (MELD) score, determined by the laboratory tests, wasn't high enough to rank him as a liver transplant candidate. "I will lose him," she told me, looking at her husband lying in the fetal position on the exam table with his eyes closed. "He doesn't believe that he'll survive. Worse, he doesn't want to survive."

Helen, who had been cheerleading for Nico and their five kids, started losing her own optimistic drive. We set up a video consultation for a second opinion from a Cleveland Clinic gastroenterologist and submitted all medical records. Less than a week later, we received a multi-page consultation report that recalculated the MELD score as high enough to rank Nico on the liver transplant list. Nico got lucky this time, and the transplant was available by the end of the month. He was a different man when I saw him a year later during the festival at the Greek Orthodox church. He was laughing and having a good time with his kids and his big Greek family.

OTHER WAYS TO MAKE DIAGNOSTIC DECISIONS

Besides expertise in their field, physicians frequently use simple algorithms that facilitate efficient and accurate decisions based on limited information called fast-and-frugal trees (FFTs). For example, ER physicians decide to admit patients with chest pain either to the Intensive Care Unit or a regular hospital bed. PCPs use fast-and-frugal tree support for prescribing antibiotics for community-acquired pneumonia or lipid-lowering medications based on the atherosclerotic cardiovascular disease (ASCVD) risk factors, for cancer screening or routinely for HIV testing and treatment. Oncologists choose types of chemotherapy based on the staging and types of cancers.[122]

Fast-and-frugal heuristics are embedded into clinical decision support algorithms in the electronic medical records, and guide clinicians in the decision-making process, to maximize correct decisions while minimizing errors. Are these shortcuts solutions for diagnostic errors? It's a help, especially in urgent situations, but not always. They can also lead to faulty clinical reasoning or conclusions.[123] Dealing with uncertainty mandates the expertise. As the Ancient Greek proverb says, "Let each man exercise the art he knows."

CHECK YOUR HEALTHCARE INVENTORY:

1. When a new diagnosis is made, seek answers to the following questions from your clinician:

    a. What makes you certain that this is the correct diagnosis?

    b. What additional testing or expert opinion do I need to confirm the diagnosis?

3. Check the list of your medical diagnoses. During your next visit with your clinician, ask:

    a. What diagnoses can be resolved?

    b. What diagnoses are lifelong?

    c. How can I reduce the risks of complications?

4. When you get a referral to a specialist, ask what criteria the referral was based on (timeliness, convenience, loyalty to a health system or hospital, expertise, outcomes). Make sure these reasons match your values.

CHAPTER 13

YOUR BODY TELLS THE STORY

Karl Hagan's face was red and moist from sweat, his gray hair was uncombed. Visibly uncomfortable and restless, he relentlessly tried to get off the gurney. Karl was heavy at 258lb and faced definite risk of fall with every turn, besides the problem that initially brought him to the ED. The appearance of two interns, upper-level residents and an attending didn't make any impression on Karl. A nurse desperately tried to calm him down. Dr. Cho, an intern, presented the patient as an 87-year-old male with a past medical history of dementia, which had worsened after his stroke three years ago, plus hypertension and coronary artery disease. Karl had been transferred from the nursing home for evaluation of fever.

Karl couldn't to speak after his last stroke, but his expression, without doubt, confirmed that he was miserable. My residents' team relied on the short note from the nursing home and the previous records from his admission for hypertensive emergency four months previously to get the medical history. Based on the nursing home note, Karl didn't have symptoms of upper respiratory infection, and no urinary symptoms of diarrhea that would give us any history clues for his current fever of 102, which he'd had for the last eight days. He was in his usual health, sitting mostly in the chair, or being in bed until he'd developed the fever and became restless.

He didn't have a history of travel, and this was before the COVID-19 pandemic. As every nursing home resident is, Karl had been tested for tuberculosis within the last six months and hadn't had any visitors within the last four weeks. Staff in the nursing home gave him Motrin and alternating Tylenol, which reduced the fever for three to four hours and made him less restless. But the symptoms relentlessly came back.

His primary care doctor had been called and prescribed a course of antibiotics, which didn't make a difference, and it was eventually suggested to take him to the ED. "His physical exam showed a temperature of 102, racing heart sounds, chronic weakness of both extremities, consistent with previous findings," summarized Dr. Cho. Blood and urine laboratory testing didn't show any clues to explain his fever, nor his chest x-ray, or CT of the abdomen and head. Labs for evaluation of autoimmune diseases and inflammatory markers were pending. When a patient gets admitted to the teaching hospital, they are evaluated by at least three physicians: the intern, an upper-level resident and then the attending physician. Residents can feel annoyed and nervous when the physician rechecks their findings.

I examined Karl and was puzzled by his "restlessness." Sometimes this can be attributed to involuntary movements, as a result of neurological changes. Watching Karl struggle, it seemed that he was trying to lift his head from the gurney. Careful exam of his face, neck, eyes with an ophthalmoscope and ears with the otoscope didn't add any value. "Can you help me to turn Karl around, I want to see his skin on the back." And there it was: three little red vesicles with yellow fluid on the back of Karl's head, close to the hairline. Karl seemed restless and wanted to move his head because of the burning pain coming from the rash from shingles.

Karl had herpes zoster-associated aseptic meningitis, a complication of herpes zoster, as his lumbar puncture confirmed. Herpes zoster is caused by the reactivation of latent varicella-zoster virus infection, the same virus that causes chicken pox. With antiviral medication and pain control, Karl finally got his rest after a few days.

What we now call a "physical exam" is actually "physical diagnosis" or diagnosis made by examination of the body. The physical diagnosis, as we know it today, has been shaped throughout the last 3,000 years. Dissections of human bodies for educational purposes began in the 13th century and led to establishing morbid anatomy, or pathology, which brought correlation of autopsy results with observational findings found by doctors at the bedside.

Modern physical diagnosis began with the localization of the disease in the patient's body with the discovery of percussion by Leopold Auenbrugger in 1760. Before Auenbrugger, physicians could not discover the location of internal disease, and diagnosis was made solely by medical history. Auenbrugger introduced the physicians' ear as a physical instrument for diagnosis—tapping body parts with fingers, hands or small instruments and listening for the produced sounds, which determined the size, consistency and borders of body organs, and the presence or absence of fluid in the body area.

Through palpation, clinicians touch and ascertain the size, consistency, texture, location, and tenderness of your organs, while auscultation helps to evaluate the sounds of the body parts (breathing, heartbeat, belly sounds, joints cracking) through listening.[124]

A physical exam is not just a diagnostic tool, it's a "hypothesis-generating tool, patient-doctor communication tool, a sign of professionalism and a stamp of clinical education," said Dr. Kurlov, while teaching us medical students the techniques of the physical exam at the Siberian State Medical University. Professor Kurlov was a short, bald man in his late 50s who wore round glasses. Dressed in a long white coat that reminded us of a magician in a cape, he spoke quietly, habitually trying not to disturb resting patients during his hospital rounds. He walked with his broad gate through the hospital corridors, his white unbuttoned robe flapping at his sides with every step, ahead of the group of students, who, like sponges, tried to pick up every pearl from this great clinician.

Dr. Kurlov was chair of the Internal Medicine Department and seemed to know all patients' stories and their diagnoses by heart. Hospital rooms on the Medicine floor were occupied by six to ten patients. We moved from one bed to another: looking, tapping, palpating bodies and listening. For us, every patient was a subject of wonder. "You have to translate the signs human bodies send into patterns, which you will build the diagnosis from," Dr. Kurlov taught. "Use all your senses: look, listen, touch and even smell to find the body's expressions of illness."

Experienced clinicians can recognize patterns of certain illnesses by visually observing the tint of skin color, skin dryness or sweat, skin tone, muscle mass, hair thickness or baldness, dilated or constricted pupils, bulging, teary or red eyes, loss of hearing, gait, posture, facial expression, voice, speed of talking, rate of breathing, muscle involvement during breathing, weight, body movements or their limitations, sadness or crying, while looking and talking to a patient in the first few minutes.

With experience, clinicians become proficient in searching and selecting illness scripts, conceptual models of groups of diseases, representational memories of specific syndromes and diagnose conditions using relatively few pieces of clinical data.[125]

"Maria, stop right there!" The assignment had been to listen to the patient's heart to recognize sounds that might give us a clue to the diagnosis. I pulled my stethoscope off the patient in fear that I'd caused harm. In a room of ten women, I imagined that the patient wouldn't be comfortable being exposed for a medical student's exam and had decided to do an auscultation through her thin, silky nightgown. Dr. Kurlov pulled me aside and said, "Can you hear variations of sound from the heart while your stethoscope's contact with the clothes generates a similar sound? How can patients rely on your knowledge of anatomy if you do not remove elements between the stethoscope and the skin that may confuse you? By listening to the heart, you have to pay attention to the timing, duration, intensity and pitch. By removing all potential obstacles between your ear and the heart, you don't just care about the right diagnosis, you show that you don't want any obstruction on the way to the diagnosis. Patients offer you their bodies so you can do your job of making a diagnosis. You must do your absolute best."

IS THE PHYSICAL EXAM STILL NECESSARY?

Rapidly advancing technology, which has introduced powerful laboratory and imaging techniques, has given us reasons to question traditional doctors' examining skills. Some clinicians start patient visits not by listening to patients' stories or examining them, but from reviewing their tests. Some, especially those who did not have extensive training in physical exams, might skip exams entirely, relying only on the test results. This approach might lead to shorter visits, but it can also lead to biased diagnosis. "It's time consuming. I can't rely on my exam alone, as I can count on the labs and tests," was the justification of one of our residents.

"Is the demise of physical diagnosis a sign of natural evolution? Did the physical exam become a fool's gold, carrying the luster of something valuable but worthless at its core?" asked Sandeep Jauhar, MD, PhD, when describing his struggles with physical exams in the article "The demise of the physical exam" published in the *New England Journal of Medicine* in 2006. He rightfully pointed out that, "Doctors today are uncomfortable with uncertainty. The fear of lawsuits is partly to blame for that, but the main culprit is the fear of subjective observation and erroneous clinical reasoning based on it."[126] Are technological shortcuts to the diagnosis justified as a modern progress of medical science and a defense from litigation?

The power of ordering the most technologically advanced tests with the highest probability of the right diagnosis is tempting. If a physical exam permits a physician to diagnose a herniated spinal disk with only 90 percent probability, then there is an almost irresistible urge to get a $1,200 MRI to close the gap.

Jim Mello was 38, an engineer, and had been physically active all his life. He jogged almost daily and coached his daughter's soccer team. "I had a cold for two weeks. It started with diarrhea and low-grade fever, then congestion and cough. All my family had the same symptoms. Everyone recovered, but I can't snap out of it." This was before the COVID-19 pandemic started. "Even minimal work makes me tired. I picked up multivitamins in the pharmacy, but they didn't change a thing. The cough got better, but I am short-winded," Jim told Dr. Brown, a third-year resident in our Family Medicine Residency Clinic.

Dr. Brown was due to graduate in two months. He didn't find anything abnormal during the exam and prescribed a short course of azithromycin, an antibiotic, thinking that Jim might have acute bronchitis. Jim called five days later to say that his shortness of breath had worsened. His chest x-ray was normal, but he had a borderline enlarged heart. Dr. Brown ordered laboratory tests thinking of pneumonia, inflammation in the lungs, and brought Jim back in. The blood test showed mildly increased white blood cells.

Dr. Lizke had joined the faculty two years before, after being a chief resident in her residency program in Boston. Attendings in the Residency Clinic serve the role of advisers to physicians in training, but they are responsible for every patient treated by residents. Something didn't make sense to her when Dr. Brown concluded that he would like to prescribe a broad-spectrum antibiotic to treat "pneumonia." He didn't say anything about the exam findings, so she went to examine the patient herself. Jim's heart was beating fast, too fast to justify his low-grade fever. "Listen to this!" she said to Dr. Brown, passing him the stethoscope. There it was—a *gallop*. Gallops can be harmless and heard in pregnant women or young athletes. In older adults, however, a gallop may indicate heart disease. Jim's gallop was an extra sound before the typical S1 systole sound, during the phase of the heartbeat when the heart muscle contracts and pumps blood from the chambers into the arteries. This sound is always indicative of a disease, likely the failure of the left ventricle of the heart.

"Let's get the electrocardiogram," (a simple test that checks the heart's rhythm and electrical activity) Dr. Lizke said. Electrocardiography showed nonspecific changes, but Jim's levels of inflammatory cardiac biomarkers were high, indicating ongoing inflammation in his heart muscle, or myocarditis. Echocardiogram, an ultrasound of the heart, with following cardiac MRI, confirmed the suspicion. The walls of Jim's heart were not moving strongly enough to squeeze the blood and push it out of the heart; a condition called cardiomyopathy.

Enteroviruses and adenoviruses, in addition to the COVID-19 virus, are the most common pathogens of viral cardiomyopathy, which people can die from if it's not treated in time. Recovery is also possible when diagnosis is made early and treatment is initiated. You notice it early by examining the patient. Jim's heart was sending SOS signals through an increased heartrate and the gallop.

Dr. Brendan Reilly, author of *One Doctor: Close Calls, Cold Cases and the Mysteries of Medicine*, conducted a study to answer the question of how important the physical exam is for making a diagnosis.[127] He compared the independent findings of physical exams made by resident-physicians and attendings in hospitalized patients, looking for parts of the physical exams that had changed the diagnosis and the plan of care. What he found was that careful physical exams changed patient diagnosis and treatment in every fourth patient. In half of these cases, the diagnostic correction was found on the physical exam and wouldn't have been discovered by "reasonable testing."

That means that testing wouldn't have been ordered if this finding wasn't discovered, unless the patient's condition worsened.

THE VALUE OF TOUCH

There is another aspect to physicians performing physical exams and that is the value of *healing touch*, which brings about the feeling of being cared for by a doctor examining a patient and putting together symptoms with exam findings. "The physical exam is a humanistic ritual that builds trust and creates the crucial bond between physician and patient—a bond that is at the core of quality health care." Said Abraham Verghese, MD, who teaches Physical Exam at Stanford University.

The power of healing touch has been recognized for centuries, not just for the skill of palpation to determine the size and features of the organs and systems, but also for healing purposes. The term *healing touch* is based on the foundation that humans have an energetic, spiritual dimension necessary for sustaining life that must be taken into account during the healing process. Healing touch is also a form of energy therapy, an alternative medicine method that is based on the belief that vital energy flows through the human body. Trained practitioners pass their hands over or gently touch to balance that energy. Healing touch therapy has been used for treatment of pain, depressive behaviors, to decrease anxiety, to increase relaxation and for a sense of wellbeing.[128]

SELF-EXAMS: TO DO OR NOT TO DO?

We see ourselves in the mirror every day and have the ability to touch, measure and monitor signals that the body sends us. But most of us don't. So, why don't people do self-exams? What if we find something? We would have to deal with it. We would rather see a doctor once a year and get a full exam. It might sound surprising but the US Preventive Services Task Force (USPSTF)—an independent, volunteer panel of national experts that creates evidence-based recommendations for preventive services—found insufficient evidence to recommend annual physical examinations of the breast, prostate, heart or anything else, concluding that the only meaningful parts of the periodic or annual physical exams are measures of vital signs (blood pressure and pulse) and body mass index, which is a person's weight in kilograms divided by the square of their height in meters. Instead, they advocated for *periodic screening*, counseling and physical exams tailored to a patient's symptoms, medical history, age, sex and risk factors.[129]

What does this mean for you? Simply, if you don't present your symptoms to your physician, or details of your history to estimate your risk, your doctor might recommend screenings, including exams, based on your age and sex, found on the USPSTF website. So, your hopes for a "full annual exam" by the doctor may not have merit, unless you provide symptoms and, together with your doctor, identify the risks. Most doctors continue the tradition of an annual full physical examination, and I am one of them. I examine my patients head to toe, trying to identify changes. When I don't find anything abnormal or changed, reassurance is a worthy result of the exam for most of my patients. Not everything in a human body is predictable, and some things are noticed accidentally, which should generate questions that otherwise would not come up. That's why the patient-doctor relationship and the art of medicine all come into play.

Is it worth examining your own body? If you're not feeling well, and come to see a doctor, the first things to be checked are your vital signs. *Vitals signs* are objective signs of the human body's condition. Based on your weight, body temperature, heartrate, respiratory rate, blood pressure and oxygen level, an impression can be made about whether your condition is "stable" or even critical.[130] If your vital signs are at the base level and within normal limits, you can feel reassured that your body seems to be okay. Clinicians use vital signs to make a diagnosis, determine if treatment is working or immediate interventions need to be made. Height and weight allow you to calculate your body mass index.[131] Obesity is an independent risk factor for heart disease, diabetes and high blood pressure. Your waist circumference can give you a quick estimate of your metabolic health.[132] By repeating measurements, you can monitor your efforts in treatments or lifestyle interventions. A thermometer, blood pressure monitor or pulse oximeter might not be the fanciest gifts, but they may save the lives of your loved ones.

The USPSTF also didn't find sufficient evidence for self-exams for screening of cancer, reminding us that the frequency of screening depends on individual risk factors and should be discussed with your clinician. Many doctors recommend checking your own skin regularly, typically once a month, especially if you have risk factors for skin cancer or a prior history of skin cancer.[133]

Although the breast self-exam technique has not been found to be reliable for breast cancer screening, 43 percent of breast cancer survivors noted that they detected breast cancers first themselves by finding a lump either by self-examination or by accident.[134] Yet there is little evidence that doing these exams routinely is helpful for women at average risk of breast cancer.[135] The American Cancer Society doesn't recommend regular clinical breast exams for cancer screening for women in any risk group. It does state, however, that all women should pay attention to the typical appearance and texture of their breasts and report any changes to their doctor right away. Techniques of breast exams for men and women are easy to learn.[136] The most important message is that a self-exam or one performed by a clinician should never substitute mammogram screening for breast cancer.

Testicular cancer can be easily detected at an early stage through self-examination. However, self-exams have also not proven to reduce the risk of dying of the disease. The American Cancer Society doesn't recommend regular testicular self-exams for all men, but we are aware that testicular cancer, if found early, can be effectively managed with simpler and less-toxic treatments.[137] Routine testicular self-exams can make you aware of the condition of your testicles and help to identify changes early.[138] I don't see any harm in doing a periodic, once-a-month self-testicular exam.

Oral health is another area that patients must watch for. Poor dental health is associated with high levels of inflammation, disability, and diabetes. It also poses a higher risk of mortality from heart disease, respiratory diseases or infections.[139] Look for gum soreness that doesn't heal, bleeding, persistent bad breath, cracked or broken teeth, teeth sensitivity and jaw pain. A dry mouth and low production of saliva was found to be associated with an increased risk of death in older men.[140] Consider your dental visits as a life-saving investment and have a dental exam at least yearly with teeth cleaning every six months, especially if you have chronic medical problems.[141]

There are testing devices that provide necessary information about chronic problems, such as a glucometer to monitor your blood sugar, or devices that measure blood coagulation (prothrombin time and international normalized ratio, PT/INR), and ovulation. We have become accustomed to doing our own pregnancy tests and COVID-19 tests. Wearable technology and transdermal biosensors are becoming more sophisticated and competitive on the market too.

The benefit of any self-exam and monitoring device is that you can monitor the signs of illness or measure certain parameters to let your clinician know about them. Your self-examination skills might be useful when you have a telemedicine visit scheduled. Measure all your vital signs before the appointment. This simple task will increase the value of your visit.

CHECK YOUR HEALTHCARE INVENTORY:

1. Go to your medicine cabinet and check what instruments you have to measure your basic vital signs: weight, blood pressure, temperature, oxygen, heartrate.

2. Based on your medical problems and risks, obtain the instruments that might be useful (pulse oximeter, blood pressure monitor, glucometer, etc.). Talk to your clinician if you have questions about the readings.

CHAPTER 14

NOT ALL TESTS ARE NECESSARY

C an you imagine telling a salesman at the car dealership, while buying a new car, "Just give me any car you recommend. I'll pay for whatever you choose." Most patients think, *If the doctor orders tests, then all the tests are necessary*. Yet, I've always wondered why patients don't ask, "Why do I need this test? Why at this time? How much does it cost? What would happen if I don't do them?"

The aftermath of unnecessary testing is much more disruptive than purchasing a vehicle that could end up in your garage to be sold later on. Unnecessary testing causes more harm than good. Futile panic and worry generated by even slightly abnormal tests will interrupt your life. Procedures, generated by false-positive tests, can end up with adverse side effects and cause pain, anxiety, time, and cost more than the benefits of the knowledge they generate.[142]

Doctors order tests to add more certainty while making medical decisions. Tests are objective findings that can quickly bring light to patients' medical dilemmas, diagnose illness in early stages and monitor treatments. Objective testing also provides reassurance for patients and confidence in the physician's judgment.[143] Most patients trust their doctor to order the right tests because doctors are trained and licensed to practice medicine, and know what tests are necessary to make a diagnosis. That is true. What is also true is that medicine is a business that uses a traditional fee-for-service reimbursement model. In this model, doctors bill for their services based on the number of requested and analyzed ancillary tests and number of medical problems diagnosed or treated. A new healthcare model, called pay for performance (P4P), or value based, provides financial incentives to practices for achieving better health outcomes. However, to determine the outcomes, many quality-based metrics require laboratory and imaging tests. The risk of being sued for the wrong diagnosis by patients also pushes physicians to order more tests, adding at least 2.4 percent of total healthcare spending.[144,145]

In 2012, the National Physicians Alliance, in partnership with the American Board of Internal Medicine, started the campaign *Choosing Wisely*®.[146] The intention was to identify the areas of inappropriate or overused tests, procedures and technologies that bring low value. Low-value care or healthcare services that do not improve patient outcomes, or for which the harm appears to outweigh the benefits, are estimated to cost the US healthcare system between $75.7 and $101.2 billion annually.[147] We talk about a low value of testing when an electrocardiogram is done for someone who has no symptoms and has a low cardiac risk, or when Pap smears are repeated every year for women with no history of abnormal Pap smears, or when a chest x-ray is done for a patient with no symptoms. These studies, done without appropriate indications, create a cascade of subsequent specialist visits, diagnostic tests, and procedures, which increase costs and provide plenty of anxiety.

HOW CAN YOU KNOW WHAT TESTS ARE NECESSARY?

First, you need to know what types of tests are available. All tests are divided into screening and diagnostic. *Screening tests* are used to determine whether you have risk factors for a particular disease compared with large numbers of seemingly healthy people. *Diagnostic tests* are used to identify an illness when symptoms are present, or screening tests have returned positive for particular conditions or risks. You can always look up the value of each test on the Choosing Wisely website.

SCREENING TESTS

A good screening test is reliable for diagnosis, meaning it's highly sensitive (or has a high probability of detecting disease) and extremely specific (or has a high probability that those without the disease will screen negative). Screening tests make a difference for an illness when treatment before symptoms occurs, which is more beneficial than after symptoms appear. For example, screening for hypertension by checking blood pressure. The earlier we start treatment of elevated blood pressure, the less the risk of cardiovascular disease and stroke. Screening of pregnant women for HIV can prevent transmission to the baby, if timely treated.

Screening tests might be an investment in your future—if you can afford them and if they are not hard to do. If a test has a high risk of adverse effects, it's simply not a good screening test. For example, cardiac catheterization will show blockages in the heart's arteries, but it cannot be done for every patient with chest pain to identify coronary artery disease. Instead, it's only done when the risks are determined to be high. From the patients' perspective, some people want to take control of their future, and some don't. Not everyone wants or can invest as much in it.

When Joanna and Richard Moore came for their wellness visit when they joined Medicare, I offered all available screening opportunities that their insurance would cover. Richard agreed to every test without asking for any details. Joanna, in contrast, had a different opinion. "I feel great. My parents lived a long life without any of those tests. At my age, of 65, whatever happens, I'll be fine with it." Richard rolled his eyes and didn't argue. Joanna died three years later from colon cancer, which was diagnosed at a late stage. She also refused any chemotherapy. Most likely, it could have been detected as a polyp and removed during screening colonoscopy, if it had been ordered. We don't know, but it was her choice.

Decisions about screening tests should be made with consideration of individual risks and certainty about the plan of action if the test is positive. Otherwise, the cost and worry about the test are not worth it. For example, certain sexually transmitted disease screening tests are justified for younger people or those with *risky* behaviors because they can be transmitted to others or when the harm from them is the highest, such as during pregnancy. Twenty years ago, we were doing Pap smears for cervical cancer screening for girls as soon as they became sexually active, even at age 16. However, studies showed that the risk of cancer was almost non-existent, especially with HPV immunizations. Now we start cervical cancer screening at age 21. We've also learned that it's not reasonable to continue either cervical cancer screening tests after the age of 65 if all prior results have been normal.[148]

The purpose of screening is to identify diseases before they happen. So, does this mean "the more the merrier"? Are ten tests better than three?

Executive physicals are offered by many of the country's largest and most respected health systems and hospitals. On a dedicated day, usually once a year, CEOs, celebrities or others who can afford it, check in to the luxury rooms, with their complimentary robes and slippers, and follow a busy agenda of testing, procedures and consultations. Among the battery of screenings that executives may be offered are often unnecessary laboratory tests, whole-body CT scans, electrocardiograms, and chest radiographs. Mostly they're an extended version of the annual physical exam that you can get in your own primary care office, with the difference of the length of time and luxurious VIP treatment.

The wealthy and privileged may be offered predictive genomics services to learn how their body uniquely metabolizes certain medications, whether they have a predisposition to specific types of disease, and whether they carry a genetic risk of disease that could be passed to their children. Testing may include stress and resilience assessments, an evaluation of cardiovascular fitness, strength, posture, balance, flexibility, and body composition. Wellness coaches offer plans for daily fitness and nutrition routines based on laboratory testing, electrocardiograms, treadmill stress tests, and pulmonary, eye and hearing tests. It's easy to understand why these elite physicals are appealing to the organizations that offer them—it is an opportunity to show off their ability to serve high-profile patients with the most advanced testing available combined with an attractive revenue stream.[149] But are they truly necessary?

Researchers from the Memorial Sloan Kettering Cancer Center, New York, analyzed executive physicals at 50 top-ranked hospitals in 43 states to see how often these physicals offered screenings and tests recommended by the USPSTF, as well as how often they included services that aren't backed by much evidence. Hearing screens and electrocardiograms, for example, which have insufficient evidence for recommendation, were offered in 83 percent of executive physicals. At the same time, none of the physicals included recommended lung cancer screenings. Many services, such as mammograms, colon cancer screening, and bone density tests, were offered as part of these physicals, even when they were only recommended for certain patient groups based on age and risk factors for specific diseases.

The benefits of resting electrocardiograms offered during elite and executive physicals for low-risk individuals haven't been backed up by existing evidence.[150] The USPSTF also warns the public that evidence is insufficient to recommend for or against testing for the ankle-brachial index (ABI), high-sensitivity C-reactive protein (hsCRP) level, or coronary artery calcium (CAC) score to traditional risk assessment for cardiovascular disease (CVD) in asymptomatic adults to prevent CVD events.[151] These tests might be beneficial in certain populations, but not as a screening for all. The conclusion of the study was that people are better off getting personalized, evidence-based care from their primary care provider, rather than an over-the-top executive physical.[152]

DIAGNOSTIC TESTS

The purpose of a diagnostic test is to establish the presence (or absence) of disease to make decisions about treatment when certain symptoms are present, or when screening tests have shown presence of illness. There are diagnostic tests that come back with definitive answers: positive or negative, such as for COVID-19, influenza, streptococcal infection, or pregnancy tests. Numeric tests come back either within or very close to the range of upper and lower limits obtained from a group of healthy people. The ranges of numeric tests might be slightly different depending on the manufacturer of the test *and* based on age, sex, sometimes race or other characteristics.

Looking at the numbers, slightly different from normal values displayed next to your results might bring extra worry. For example, the average hemoglobin and hematocrit levels, white blood cell count and absolute granulocyte count normal values for African Americans can be slightly lower than for Caucasians.[153] There are substantial ethnic differences in bone mineral densities between African or Asian individuals, which have to be accounted for when interpreting values of fracture risks among postmenopausal women screenings.[154] Ask your clinician the question of whether your results are comparable with normal limits for someone your age and ethnicity to avoid anxiety and repeating the test.

TESTING CASCADE

When patients have ambiguous complaints, which could be caused by a multitude of clinical conditions (I feel tired, my energy level is low), physicians might use a "shotgun approach" (a barrage of tests), instead of focusing on the important elements of history or exam. Ordering multiple tests or tests that have low value may bring a lot of surprising findings that will be difficult to explain and, most importantly, act upon. As a result, clinicians will order more tests and procedures.[155]

Karen Wittik, a registered nurse, requested a cancer antigen 125 (CA-125) test—a tumor marker for ovarian cancer—to be checked among other tests to find the reasons for her fatigue. "I had an ovarian cyst in the past and wanted to make sure I didn't have ovarian cancer." Sometimes, it's hard to argue, especially with our medical professional colleagues, and I am guilty of taking their side more than I should. The test came back moderately elevated. It started a chain of imaging tests, all of which were negative. Karen's anxiety was through the roof, and she underwent a laparoscopy—a surgical procedure where a fiber-optic instrument is inserted through the abdominal wall to view the organs and get a biopsy. This also failed to find ovarian cancer. The normal results of all these tests didn't bring reassurance to Karen, who lost her peace for years and continued rechecking the CA-125, searching for cancers. If you look at the Choosing Wisely website, CA-125 is not a good test for low-risk women. It may be helpful for women with a known high risk of developing ovarian cancer, or women with known ovarian cancer, to monitor treatment and watch for recurrence[156]. High CA-125 false-positive results have been noted in many medical disorders, both malignant and benign, because CA-125 is known to have poor sensitivity and specificity.[157]

Questions about testing require decisions to be made while ordering, performing tests and communicating results to assure that tests will bring certainty and guide your health outcomes.

CHECK YOUR HEALTHCARE INVENTORY:

Ask the following questions when tests are ordered:

1. Why is the test being ordered?

2. What is the cost, and will it be covered by my insurance?

3. Are there alternative laboratories where costs might be less prohibitive?

4. How do I get the results and an explanation of them?

CHAPTER 15

TOO MUCH MEDICINE, TOO LITTLE CARE

Jury Aliev, one of my Russian patients, came in with chest and left arm pain, which happened to be a recurrent thing recently. The pain had become constant but didn't get worse with exertion. Jury was a barber, who in his previous Russian life was a chemist and taught chemistry in the Polytechnical Institute in Tashkent before he immigrated to the USA with his extended family. In his 60s, slightly overweight, with curly, balding hair, Jury made me laugh out loud with his endless jokes. My exam didn't reveal any abnormal findings, which is common in patients with heart disease, which I worried about in "60-year-old overweight male with chest pain."

His EKG didn't show any dangerous signs, but I couldn't hold myself back from running through his risk factors, which seemed to be on the low side. I found his recent chest x-ray, which was normal. My first intention was to send Jury to the ED for cardiac evaluation. But Jury had a different plan in mind.

"Try to do this dance every day, Doc," he said, noticing my puzzled look. He stood up, lifted his arms, the left arm a little lower than the right, and started making circular motions with his wrists to a familiar Russian melody that he produced to accompany his barber "dance." A smile immediately came to my face instead of worry.

I saw him standing in this position with the comb in the left hand and scissors in the right for hours. "I think it's my back that needs some love and care, Doc. Trust me." He did have tenderness next to his thoracic spine line on the left side, so Jury promised to go to the ER if the pain got worse and agreed to go for physical therapy, use a TENs unit (a machine that delivers small electrical impulses to the affected area to relieve pain and relax muscles) and topical treatments for his upper back. The pain was gone in four weeks.

My plan was to send Jury to the ER for evaluation of his chest pain, which could be a sign of angina or tearing aorta. Instead, I had to do something more difficult: trust my patient and hope that he knew his body better than me. I told Jury about my concerns about potential tragic outcomes if no interventions were made. He listened carefully, smiled, and said, "Don't worry, Doc. I will be fine." Shared decision-making is one of the ways to mitigate overtreatment.

WHAT IS OVERTREATMENT?

When the interventions don't change the health outcome or benefit the patient, or where the risk of harm from the intervention is likely to outweigh the expected benefits, we call it overtreatment. It may be classed as *overuse* of medical services when interventions are not necessary, or *over-testing*, when tests wouldn't change the management of the medical condition. It also might be an *overdiagnosis* when we label symptoms or signs that are non-threatening, non-progressive or even improving, and will not affect the person's quality of life or don't have to be treated.[158] A perception that more care results in a better outcome happens to be a myth, according to the research.[159]

Biopsy of skin lesions that haven't changed over time and look benign is an example of overdiagnosis, as well as a colonoscopy performed for a 78-year-old person who doesn't have gastroenterological symptoms but is suffering with respiratory and heart problems.

The patient may end up with serious complications from anesthesia or a GI bleed without the actual benefit of knowing that everything is well in the colon. Ordering an electrocardiogram on a healthy 50-year-old without symptoms, just to "check their heart," is over-testing and has no benefits.

Overtreatment is not good for patients or doctors. The more tests a doctor orders, the more abnormal results will come back, triggering more tests and unnecessary treatments. With overtreatment comes extra hardship for doctors as well as medical offices, with more results to follow up, more appointments to schedule and pre-authorize with insurance companies. All of which distract physicians and staff from more meaningful patient care.

If this isn't good for patients and doctors, why do unnecessary healthcare services account for close to 25 percent of total US health-care spending, or $760 billion to $935 billion each year?[160]

Being a part of academic medicine for more than three decades, I am guilty of training young physicians "diligence," or thorough workup of medical problems. In medical schools, students are encouraged to get to the bottom of the medical problem, sometimes without looking at the cost because *lives are at stake*. During graduate training, residents' confidence is low, and experience limited, so over-treatment can be confused with comprehensiveness with the intention of high-quality patient care. This intention sometimes leads to forming habits of overworking symptoms and problems that can't be changed or treated.

Practicing habits learned during residency can stay for a long time. Less-experienced physicians who have been trained in high-spending practices, continue the same spending pattern after training, while more experienced physicians traditionally spend less.[161]

Physicians are in the position of balancing between undertreatment and overtreatment. Both are examples of suboptimal care and can harm.[162] We have the best intentions in mind while getting blood sugar and blood pressure under control in patients with diabetes or hypertension. When we go too far and lower blood sugar and blood pressure too low, both interventions can be harmful for patients with heart disease, causing more complications than benefits. Prescribing multiple medications by different specialists for good reasons may lead to interactions between the medications and an increased potential for side effects. Instead of working closely with patients on behavior change to lose weight or improve sleep, which takes more time, we succumb to the habit of prescribing more medications.

Antibiotic misuse has led to the development of bacterial and antibiotic resistance. An overuse of unnecessary screenings, such as Pap smears for women over 65 years old without a history of abnormal Pap smears, or screening colonoscopies in the elderly, which exposes patients to risks, triggers unnecessary procedures. End of life is an area where overtreatment reaches the ceiling, with one-third of adults undergoing procedures with no clinical or palliative benefit during their last six months of life.[163]

WHY DO DOCTORS OVERTREAT?

Researchers from Harvard Medical School and Johns Hopkins University School of Medicine interviewed 2,106 physicians about the necessity of their medical care. More than 20 percent of them offered unnecessary services, including every fifth prescription medication and test, and every tenth procedure. The number-one reason was doctors' fear of malpractice, followed by patient pressure, and difficulty accessing medical records.[164] Financial incentives for overtreatment are small in comparison with the physician's intention to be comprehensive and provide high-quality patient care. It feels more comforting to order higher-probability tests and it is tempting to do more rather than less.[165]

One of the powerful forces driving overtreatment is the patients themselves. We fall for advertised "miracle" drugs and super-effective medical treatments the same as new shoes. Sugar-loaded drinks end up on our tables under the pretense of providing "vitamins and energy." Pharmaceutical advertisements frequently omit facts or downplay risks, overstate a drug's benefits, make claims that are not appropriately supported and have misleading drug comparisons, fooling patients into asking doctors to prescribe them instead of the old-fashioned, proven to be effective and not expensive remedies and treatments.

Semaglutide, or Ozempic, produced by the drug manufacturer Novo Nordisk for treatment of diabetes, became famous for its weight-loss properties, which first made headlines in 2021 from *The Dr. Oz Show* in a segment titled, "Could a Diabetes Drug Cure Obesity?" A higher dose of Ozempic's active ingredient, semaglutide 2.4mg, was approved for weight loss in June 2021 under the name Wegovy. The cost of Wegovy before insurance is around $1,400 a month, and Ozempic's out-of-pocket rate is around $900 a month. People become fascinated by social media and its ability to make celebrities "fit, ripped and healthy." On TikTok, the hashtag #Ozempic has been viewed over 273 million times.[166] Not surprisingly, people started asking for Ozempic off-label prescriptions, as a quick fix for weight loss in a short timeframe.

Common examples of overtreatment are costly MRIs and computerized tomography (CT) scans, which are increasingly being ordered for routine low back pain (LBP). More than 85 percent of us will have uncomplicated LBP at some point, which usually improves within a few weeks without significant interventions and doesn't warrant evaluation with any imaging.[167] Typical imaging findings, such as disk degeneration, facet arthropathy and disk herniations, attributed to LBP, have been found in a large proportion of asymptomatic individuals with aging. They are going to be there just as wrinkles are expected to be seen more or less when we age. An MRI is highly sensitive and will detect all degenerative changes in the spine, but it doesn't mean that those changes are responsible for the present LBP or should drive decision-making about the treatments.[168] It's a different story if advanced imaging such as CT and MRI are used in patients with radiculopathy that doesn't respond to conservative management, myelopathy, neurogenic claudication, or patients with "red flag" symptoms.

WHAT CAN YOU DO TO PREVENT OVERTREATMENT?

I would put my money into one strategy: collaborative decisions made by a patient and a doctor. A relationship that frees up the patient's expression of their own opinions, values, and trust to the doctor, who also returns that trust to the patient by delivering as much information as possible in an understandable format. Our role as patients is to deliberate our values and concerns with the physician's opinion. When the National Physicians Alliance, in partnership with the American Board of Internal Medicine, started the campaign Choosing Wisely®,[169] the intention was to identify the areas of inappropriate or overused procedures and technologies that bring no value. The low-risk diagnostic tests and treatments can befound on Choosing wisely website or the app.

What frequently happens is that we either leave the doctor's office and don't follow the advice, which may lead to the progression of symptoms or complications of illness, or we blindly follow medical advice without expressing our opinion, which could have cut down the number of ordered tests and unnecessary treatments. Clinicians don't always invite patients to share medical decisions, but *you don't have to wait for an invitation*. Start the conversation, and change clinicians, if necessary, to someone who will listen to you and respect your values.

CHECK YOUR HEALTHCARE INVENTORY:

1. When a test or treatment has been prescribed to you, did you ask your clinician why this particular method is the best option? Are there alternatives?

2. Check two of the most recent treatments prescribed to you on the Choosing Wisely® website.

CHAPTER 16

A PILL FOR EVERYTHING

The US carries the name of "pill nation" as we believe there is a pill for everything: weight loss, a happy mood, productivity, pain, memory… More than half of adults in the US regularly take, on average, four prescription medications. Two-thirds of Americans take at least one over-the-counter medication in addition to prescription meds.[170] An estimated $200 billion per year is spent in the US on the unnecessary and improper use of medications, for the drugs themselves and related medical costs.[171] Do we always know the real issue, or do we try to hide behind the short fix of one or more supplements or prescription medications? If, through taking a pill, we can solve the problem, instead of exercising, not eating our favorite foods, or figuring out the personal life issues that bring us stress, why not?

The purpose of any medication is to change human body functions that have failed, or to treat or prevent illness. The human body is a complicated machine, where different functions are interconnected. Changing one functionality affects others. Not every medication might work for everyone, and there is always the risk of a harmful interaction between the medicine and a food, dietary supplement or another medicine. The challenge is to balance the benefits and risks of medication while trying to achieve the desired effect and catch the unwelcome adverse reactions. Patients count on doctors for these tasks, but in real life, most of the time doctors get involved when the side effects or medical errors have already happened.

It was close to lunchtime and our last patient, a lovely 78-year-old, Lucy Cavanaugh, closed the door of the clinic and was limping slowly to her car in the parking lot. Dressed in a loose pink shirt and wide white pants with white sneakers and a wide-brimmed straw hat, Lucy was putting a lot of pressure on the cane she held in her right hand, holding her bright-red purse in her left.

"Did we make the right decision not sending Lucy to the ED for evaluation?" asked Dr. July Abbot, our graduating family medicine resident, who was looking at Lucy through the big window of the precepting room. At noon on weekdays, faculty and attendings got together for a lecture while eating lunch or drinking a cup of coffee. Noon lectures at the residency program weren't just a chance to get more knowledge, but were a way to communicate with each other, share interesting cases and updates about mutual patients. That sunny day, our lecturer hadn't shown up. The weather was beautiful, and we decided to grab a quick lunch in the Vietnamese restaurant across the street. "You might be right," I said, after taking another glimpse at Lucy, who was sluggishly opening the shiny door of her Buick.

Lucy had been a patient in the Residency Clinic for years. She proudly used to say, "I raised all those doctors," while chatting with other seniors invited for yearly holiday lunches to celebrate Thanksgiving and Christmas. The patients' appreciation lunches, thrown by residents and faculty, became a tradition in our residency program and were supported by the affiliated community hospital. Our senior patients loved to meet their doctors around the big table for a traditional Thanksgiving meal. It created a special bond that brought the patient-doctor relationship to a new level.

Lucy's house was just a few miles away, and she was thankful for her independence, living alone at her age. Her only son lived 3,000 miles away "up north" and Lucy had no desire to leave her beloved

South, where she was born and raised. She volunteered in the same church where she'd sung in the chorus when she was a little girl, and she visited her girlfriends for a weekly game of bridge.

This morning, Lucy had called and asked to be seen: "I feel woozy." Dizziness is a common problem in the elderly and can be a symptom of numerous diseases. Lucy had rheumatoid arthritis and took medications for the pain in her knees, hips, and fingers. Her medication list was not as extensive as that of some of our other elderly patients but included six other medications she took for diabetes, blood pressure and cholesterol.

Dr. Abbot, her doctor, was a favorite among the elders. She knew her patients by their first names, remembered their hobbies and seemed interested in all updates about neighbors, children, and grandchildren. Lucy asked her doctor about the preparation for her upcoming wedding, concluding, "You'll be gorgeous no matter what you wear."

"Are you dizzy only when you stand up, or change your position?" Dr. Abbot asked.

"I don't know, I feel it all the time. I feel more tired than dizzy, but I never pass out and don't feel I'm about to. Just unsteady, I guess."

"I see you've been taking the same medications as we prescribed. Any chance you might have forgotten some over-the-counter medications?"

"Well, I take Tylenol for pain at night. It should be in my records."

"It wasn't in the records, but will be now," reassured Dr. Abbot.

"I saw my rheumatologist last month. He said he'd let you know. He gave me a 'little yellow capsule'. It should be in the records." Lucy felt upset that her doctor didn't know about her visit to the rheumatologist and the new medication prescribed.

INFORMATION EXCHANGE

Patients expect doctors to do their homework and look up the previous records before their visit without realizing that medical records from different practices don't always communicate. Doctors might not be aware about the medications that have been prescribed or discontinued by another physician.

Interoperability of EMR systems has been a challenge in healthcare for decades. Different EMR platforms don't talk to each other unless special interfaces are created. In 2018 from 571,045 providers affiliated with 4,023 hospitals, there were 16 different EMR platforms used in hospitals and medical offices.[172] This is in addition to internal EMR systems created and owned by individual medical groups.

So, what does this mean for patients? Offices and hospitals, unless they share the same medical records platforms, are not aware about patients' histories, test results, medications or procedures. In 2018, every third patient who went to a doctor experienced a gap in health information exchange. One out of five patients had to redo a test or procedure or provide health information because their prior data was unavailable.[173] Large EMR vendors, like EPIC or Cerner, have created opportunities to retrieve individuals' data from other health systems who use the same platform. Otherwise, to overcome this unsolved healthcare problem, patients have no other option but to meticulously keep their own records in paper or electronic forms.

Dr. Abbot called Lucy's pharmacy and found out that her rheumatologist had prescribed *gabapentin* to help with pain, which had a side effect of dizziness. Lucy's physical exam didn't reveal any new findings to explain her symptoms, but mild edema of both legs. The electrocardiogram tracing of her heart also didn't show any new changes. We ordered additional bloodwork to check for other reasons that could contribute to dizziness and leg swelling and planned to check on her the next day, warning Lucy to call 911 if she was feeling worse. Dr. Abbot suspected it was the gabapentin that had contributed to the dizziness and asked Lucy to reduce its dose. Lucy assured us she felt well while leaving the clinic.

As soon as we started crossing the road towards the restaurant where we planned to have lunch, Dr. Abbot pushed me back. "Wait." She saw Lucy's car had backed off from the parking spot and was making slow moves toward the major road. She rushed toward the car and started banging on the driver's window. Even through the window, we could see Lucy's sleepy and pale face. We called 911.

That's when you remember that you have to trust the little voice that tells you to send a patient to the hospital for evaluation instead of letting them go home. After multiple diagnostic tests, our inpatient team didn't find any other causes for Lucy's dizziness but the new medication. The doctors also asked to look at all medications that Lucy was actually taking. In her bag was Tylenol PM, which has two medications in it: acetaminophen and diphenhydramine. The latter has the side effect of somnolence and dizziness. Interaction between gabapentin and diphenhydramine, both medications with similar side effects, was the reason for Lucy's somnolence and dizziness.

Every medication comes with some side effects. As we age, the number of medications we take often grows with the number of medical problems we have, as well as the risk of interactions between them and risk of side effects. In 1991, Dr. Mark Beers, a geriatrician, created the first list of potentially harmful medications for older adults, which was later adapted as an expert-based guidance for prescribing medications for the elderly.[174] Diphenhydramine (Benadryl), frequently considered harmless to the younger individual, and which can be purchased in the local pharmacy without prescription, is on the Beer's list as a potentially harmful medication to be avoided. Lucy told her doctors that she was taking Tylenol, but it was actually Tylenol PM, which has diphenhydramine in it.

According to one consumer poll, only one-third of the public could identify the active ingredient in their brand of pain reliever.[175] Researchers from the University of Chicago and Johns Hopkins University estimated that 70 percent of elders take supplements and OTC medications together with prescribed medications. As a result, approximately one in six older adults may be at risk for a major drug-drug interaction.[176] Patients have to deal with complexities of pharmacology and healthcare delivery missteps every time medications are prescribed. If Lucy had told the doctor that she was taking Tylenol PM, and not just Tylenol, the interaction would have been detected by the EMR software at the time it was prescribed. Fortunately, Lucy was back to her "independent" life and both the gabapentin and Tylenol PM were stopped. We can't blame patients for their lack of knowledge, but we ask that you bring a detailed list of all medications you take, including over the counter, with you to every visit.

ARE YOU TAKING ENERGY ZAPPERS?

Fatigue or "low energy" is one of the most common complaints in primary care.[177] It might come out as "I feel exhausted," "I'm stressed out," "I can't take it anymore," "Everything hurts," or, "I can't live like that." When men present with fatigue, they typically complain of "feeling tired." Women tend to describe fatigue as feeling "depressed or anxious."[178] Fatigue disrupts work performance, quality of life, family, and social relationships. According to a 2018 National Safety Council survey report, two-thirds of the US labor force, which means close to 107 million people, feel tired and exhausted at the workplace. Fatigue has multiple dimensions, with links to stress, pain, and inflammation, and is difficult to avoid and control. Fatigue is also one of the most common side effects of multiple medications and the results of interactions between them.

The list of prescription medications commonly associated with fatigue and drowsiness side effects is long and extensive:

- Antihistamines
- Antidepressants
- Anxiety medications

- Blood pressure meds
- Gastrointestinal medications to control nausea and vomiting
- Antibiotics (especially the commonly used ones: azithromycin, amoxicillin, Augmentin, penicillin)
- Cancer treatments
- Muscle relaxants
- Pain medications
- Seizure and epilepsy medications
- Medications for Parkinson's disease
- Anti-itching medications
- Corticosteroids
- Certain anti-rheumatological drugs (DMARDs)

You name it and it's on the list! It does not mean that you have to stop taking your medications. Be mindful and discuss potential side effects and timing when you have to take your medications with your clinician.

Medications are one of the top five reasons for drowsy or fatigued driving, and 328,000 drowsy driving crashes occur annually.[179]

Dr. Steve Cary, one of my colleagues from the hospital, wasn't a frequent flier in the clinic. I saw him mostly for injuries as a result of his active lifestyle, which he continued into his 60s. Doctors don't like to talk about weight, unless it's about transformational weight loss—another sign of success. The last time I'd seen Steve was about eight months before, after his ankle fracture. Steve had clearly put on some weight and was limping when I passed him at the hospital. "Still hurts?" I asked. He nodded his head in agreement. Steve hadn't been able to regain his active lifestyle after that ankle fracture, which he had chosen not to operate on: "I don't have time for surgery. It'll heal, not a big deal," he'd decided.

He started using OTC Aleve and Motrin—non-steroidal anti-inflammatory drugs (NSAIDs)—almost daily to alleviate the pain that never went away. After a few months, he felt more tired. When he eventually came into the clinic to have the swelling of both ankles checked, the laboratory results showed signs of anemia (decreased amount of healthy red blood cells that carry adequate oxygen to the body) and signs of renal impairment.

NSAIDs, sold as Ibuprofen (Advil, Motrin) and Naproxen (Aleve, Anaprox DS, Naprosyn), relieve pain and fever. People keep them handy in cars, purses and office drawers. The mechanism of these drugs is based on blocking the enzyme called *cyclooxygenase*. This is produced during tissue injury and is linked to the production of prostaglandins—hormone-like substances that control inflammation, blood flow and clot formation, contracting or relaxing smooth muscles in the uterus and gastrointestinal tract, opening or closing airways, and decreasing eye pressure. Prostaglandins promote pain reduction, but they can also cause it.

When taken for months instead of occasional use, NSAIDs reduce the inflammatory response but at the expense of energy stores, in addition to potential daily headaches and other side effects from peptic ulcers to renal failure and photosensitivity.

Stories like Steve's are common. We often read about potential side effects but hope they won't happen and continue taking OTC medications for a long time without discussing them with clinicians, counting on their safety. "If medications are freely available without prescription, they are safe," is our rationale. They might be safe for a short period but are not intended to be taken for a long time, which is usually written in the warning label.

Unfortunately, only one in five Americans read warning information when buying OTC drugs. One-third say they take more than the recommended dose of a non-prescription medicine, believing that it will increase the effectiveness of the product. Sixty-three percent report taking the next dose sooner than directed, and almost half say they take more than the recommended number of doses in a day.[180]

When you take OTC medication, you act as your own doctor. It comes with the responsibility of knowing the side effects of every medication or supplement, interactions with food or other medications you're already taking and time limits. Read the label and follow the instructions.

MEDICATIONS ARE NOT
YOUR LIFELONG COMPANIONS

Dave Gleason was 62 when I met him. He loved jogging at least four to five times a week and attended a gym frequently. Food was his passion—he was a great cook and had mastered international cuisines, which he proudly talked about. He sailed his 36-foot boat all over the world and enjoyed his early retirement. Dave took two medications to control his blood pressure, one medication for high cholesterol, two for arthritis and one for gastroesophageal reflux. Dave didn't have a primary care doctor and preferred to be treated by specialists. He visited a cardiologist for his high blood pressure and cholesterol, a gastroenterologist and orthopedist once a year to manage his chronic conditions. He felt well and all his medical problems had been under control for years. "Don't rock the boat; this regimen works well for me," he warned every doctor he had seen.

He improved his diet, lost some weight and his blood pressure was persistently below 110/70, but Dave continued to take two blood pressure medications, happy about the successful treatment. He'd reduced foods that caused his reflux symptoms, including his favorite tomatoes and chili, which he now only cooked two or three times a year. But he was also committed to taking Prilosec because, "If I don't, the heartburn will probably come back."

Dave came to our Primary Care Clinic after his second episode of pneumonia, which came as a surprise. He'd never smoked or had respiratory issues. During hospitalization, it was discovered that he had declining renal function and he was referred to a kidney specialist, who assured him that his kidneys looked good on the ultrasound, but there were "chronic changes contributing to chronic kidney disease." After multiple tests, no other significant reasons for kidney disease were found. The nephrologist concluded that most likely his stage 3 chronic renal disease was caused by the side effects of Motrin and omeprazole that he'd continuously taken for the last 15 years, and persistently low blood pressure. Vitamin D and alendronate were prescribed for osteoporosis, found on the bone density scan. Vitamin B12 was added for severe B12 deficiency.

"Why did this all happen? I've seen my doctors regularly." What happened to Dave is called "polypharmacy cascade." Dave's lifestyle and low-salt, whole-food diet had helped to normalize his blood pressure. Two blood pressure medications brought his blood pressure to unnecessarily low targets, decreasing blood flow to his kidneys and together, with the regular use of NSAIDs, contributed to poor renal function.[181]

Proton pump inhibitors are powerful and effective drugs when used for the right reasons with the lowest effective dose to treat peptic ulcer disease, dyspepsia, GERD, Barrett's esophagus, esophagitis, and other conditions that would benefit from decreased hydrochloric acid in the stomach. Unfortunately, 70 percent of people use them without an appropriate indication, being unaware of the multiple long-term adverse effects described in the observation studies: bone fractures, kidney diseases, memory loss, low magnesium levels, B12 deficiency, pneumonia, and colitis.[182,183] Dave's kidneys took a hit from three different groups of medications.

Among those who take prescription medications, the average number of medications taken is four. Almost half of seniors take five or more medications. Up to 91 percent of patients in long-term care take at least five medications daily. Younger adults with chronic pain, fibromyalgia or with developmental disabilities, patients with diabetes, heart disease, stroke and cancer are at risk for polypharmacy cascade.[184] The reasons are several: doctors of different specialties prescribe different treatment modalities; complexity of diseases; and disintegrated medical records.

It's much easier for physicians to prescribe medication than to convince patients to stop medication that they have been taking for years, sometimes decades, and which have become unnecessary.

De-prescribing is the reducing or discontinuing of medications that aren't necessary, have risks that outweigh the benefits, interact with other more important medications or can simply cause harm. Medications change your bodily functions. When these have been changed with medication, the body adapts to a certain level of functioning. Abrupt quitting of a medication can not only bring the symptoms back, it can also be followed by dangerous withdrawal symptoms, as could happen with antidepressants, clonidine and propranolol, medications that are prescribed for blood pressure treatment, and benzodiazepines. As with prescribing medications, de-prescribing must be done carefully by a physician.

Medications are not your lifelong companions. The principle "the more the merrier" does not work here. The more medications you take, the more risks of side effects and interactions you will be exposed to. If you take medications for chronic illnesses, learn what every medication is for, how long you have to take each one and how safe they are for long-term use. If you see specialists who prescribe you certain medications, don't have an expectation that they will adjust your other medications. The best place to go through all your medications and ensure that they don't interact with each other, and that you aren't experiencing side effects, is your primary care doctor's office. Start the conversation about "de-prescribing."

CHECK YOUR HEALTHCARE INVENTORY:

1. Make a list of all prescribed and over-the-counter medications that you take. Make sure you are aware what each medication is for and how long you should be taking it.

2. During your next visit, discuss and write down the potential side effects, interactions and expected length of treatment for all your medications. Are there any medications that could be de-prescribed?

CHAPTER 17

THE REALITY OF DIETARY SUPPLEMENTS

When I experienced the side effects of a medication prescribed to me to improve my heart function and reduce stress, as many of my patients do, I started searching for alternative options. Almost half of Americans take dietary supplements[185] for overall wellness, heart health, nutritional benefits, to improve immune function and energy levels, sleep and sexual performance, enhance memory, reduce stress, and lose weight. According to consumer surveys, most of us believe that supplements are good for our health and wellness, and 61 percent trust supplements to treat colds. Every second person surveyed had considered supplements for arthritis, depression, and influenza.[186]

One-third of those interviewed considered dietary supplements helpful in the treatment of cancer.[187] This is a troublesome statistic! The American Institute for Cancer Research has recommended against the use of dietary supplements for cancer prevention because of the unpredictability of the potential benefits and risks, as well as the possibility of unexpected adverse events.[188] One of the points of view is that the use of antioxidant dietary supplements by cancer patients undergoing treatment might slow down the effect of therapy because many chemotherapy drugs rely on oxidation to induce cell death. That's why the National Cancer Institute recommends that people who are being treated for cancer talk with their oncologist before taking any supplements.

The reality is that only one-third of people discuss their supplement use with physicians.[189,190,191] Without a doubt, people are taking the doctoring torch into their own hands, accepting the risks of delaying diagnosis and the use of proven, effective treatments or using supplements for a potentially wrong diagnosis. So, why are we so ready to believe in the miracles of dietary supplements? Could it be because information about dietary supplements is easily available on the internet, and they are easy to buy?

SUPPLEMENTS EFFICACY

It's hard to say whether dietary supplements are effective for the symptoms symptoms you are aiming for. One of the reasons for that is the difficulty in proving causation of either their efficacy or side effects based on reports without well-conducted, randomized clinical trials. Conventional wisdom from the randomized, controlled studies done on medications makes physicians feel safe while prescribing them. Randomized trials and any detailed research require millions of dollars to prove efficacy and safety. It is unrealistic to expect the same level of investment or research into dietary supplements, which are produced by many different manufacturers, and it also may take a longer time to reach similar effects to prescribed medications. Non-patentable herbs are not a research priority, are done on small samples of participants and are not financially feasible.[192] The safety of dietary supplements is also easily misunderstood. We tend to have a false sense of security while using supplements made from natural substances. Some of us also falsely consider supplements as "magic bullets" that are natural and safe, and we find a lot of positives in taking easily available, without a prescription and less-expensive supplements.[193] While dietary supplements are not intended to treat illnesses, we have false hopes that they are "safe" alternatives for the treatment of chronic illnesses.

One example was Rosalie Sanders, with her lifelong mission to lose weight. She was 32 years old and slightly overweight, which she blamed her hypothyroidism (underactive thyroid) for, despite her thyroid's reduced function being controlled on daily levothyroxine. Rosalie had tried all kinds of remedies she found on the internet. This time she scheduled an appointment in the clinic for "belly pain."

"You should be proud of me, I finally lost weight. It's all natural. I do eat a ton of fruits and vegetables," she said. Rosalie looked happy after losing almost 15lb in three months but was worried about abdominal cramps, loose stools, and itching. Her exam was completely normal, but her skin was an unusually bright pink/red and dry in the sun-exposed areas.

Rosalie's laboratory tests came back normal, but her thyroid function was off, despite her usual daily supplementation with levothyroxine, which she had been taking for years. The acute onset of skin irritations, abdominal cramps, and diarrhea with a 15lb weight loss could be the pattern of multiple diseases, including inflammatory bowel disease. "I'm so happy I found the way to lose weight," replied Rosalie in response to my concerns about her unexplained diarrhea and abdominal cramping. I proposed a referral to a gastroenterologist. We also adjusted the dose of her thyroid supplementation medication. I asked Rosalie to keep a journal of her abdominal cramps and heartburn for a week, paying attention to what food she ate a few hours prior.

After we reviewed the journal, it became clear that her abdominal cramps and bloating came up 30–45 minutes after she drank her smoothie.

"Tell me more about this smoothie," I said.

"I want to lose more weight before the vacation, so I drink the smoothie twice a day."

"What's in the smoothie?"

"Just a natural celery powder I bought from this website," she said, pulling it up on her phone. "Plus, I added a few stalks of fresh kale, lettuce, and ice cubes. I've eaten celery before, but mostly cooked in chili or soups, and never experienced any symptoms," she said, trying to convince me.

Multiple websites that Rosalie went to claimed the weight-loss benefits of celery, as well as for sleep and even joint pain from gout and rheumatoid arthritis. One large stalk of celery contains only ten calories, with a high percentage of that being water and fiber. If substituted for high-caloric meals, it could create benefits for weight loss simply through caloric restriction. What many people don't know is that in large amounts, celery powder can increase skin sensitivity to the sun due to photosensitizing agents such as phenols and psoralens, and this was the reason for Rosalie's dry and burned skin. Celery in large amounts as a powder can also interfere with thyroid medication.[194]

As a result, Rosalie's usual dose of levothyroxine had become too high and promoted more weight loss. Celery juice is high in insoluble fiber or FODMAPs (fermentable monosaccharides, oligosaccharides, disaccharides, and polyols, which are short-chain carbohydrates (sugars) that your body has difficulty digesting). It can feed bacteria in the gut with symptoms of gas, bloating and pain in the digestive tract. After Rosalie eliminated her "miracle weight-loss powder" remedy for a month, as you might guess, her symptoms were gone, and her thyroid tests returned to normal on the previous dose of her levothyroxine.

The three main categories of supplements prone to the most adverse side effects are those for sexual enhancement, weight loss and sports performance/bodybuilding. However, there are other aspects that may question supplement safety, related to how they are being used.

My conversations with patients about using supplements typically start with their expressed desire to take "natural" products, instead of medications, with the assumption that "medications are chemicals bearing more harm, while natural products are safe."

However, one of my biggest concerns is that by taking supplements instead of medications, we allow illnesses to progress and complications to develop. Almost 23 million Americans reported using dietary supplements instead of prescription medications.[195]

So, this question of supplement efficacy cannot be answered without discussion with your clinician about your symptoms, illness diagnosis, potential interactions, and related risks. In the situations when diagnosis is established and the risks are low (for example, cold, irritable bowel syndrome, migraine) a time-framed trial of dietary supplements can be considered.

MISINTERPRETATION

I see a lot of confusion between the doses of supplements—and the effects of concentrated or combined supplements packed in a capsule or tincture—being misinterpreted with their individual benefits. Being mindful about supplements means being aware not only about the correct doses and length of use, but also of the preparations, brands, and reliable manufacturers. Not everyone understands that doses of supplements are also highly specific, just as doses of medications are, with the difference that supplements are not intended to change one body functionality. Most of the time they affect many body systems and therefore are best used from starting "low" and moving "slow," while watching the effects and titrating as needed.

However, even supplements can have side effects, though they are measured on a much lesser scale than prescription drugs. The 2013 Annual Report of the American Association of Poison Control Centers revealed 1,692 fatalities due to drugs, and zero deaths due to supplements. Less than one percent of Americans experience adverse events related to supplements, and the majority were classified as minor, with many of these related to caffeine, yohimbe or other stimulant ingredients. The number-one "offender" in dietary supplements is drugs, followed by new dietary ingredients that have not been submitted to the FDA—both are illegal and are not dietary supplements, but, rather, "tainted products marketed as dietary supplements."

Multivitamins (MVMs) deserve a special word in the discussion of dietary supplements. Every third American takes MVMs, contributing to the growing $5.7 billion MVM industry. Among long-term cancer survivors, use of vitamin or mineral supplements is even higher at 64–81 percent.[196] Not everyone is aware that all MVMs are not the same. Manufacturers determine the types and levels of all ingredients in their MVMs, frequently focusing on specific needs of children, adults, men, women, pregnant women, and seniors. As a result, many types of MVMs are available on the market. Some of them may include other nutritional products (for example, sterols, coenzyme Q10, probiotics and glucosamine) and herbal ingredients for specific targets on energy, memory, stress relief, weight control, immune function, or management of menopausal symptoms.

What makes it more complicated is that manufacturers might label a product containing several vitamins, minerals, amino acids, and herbs as a "stress relief booster" or an "immune formula" rather than an MVM, even though it contains several vitamins and minerals. Some consider taking MVMs as nutritional insurance; a concept first introduced by Miles Laboratories in marketing its One-A-Day line of supplements. If you are an adult without nutritional deficiencies, there is no benefit in taking vitamin and mineral supplements, which has been confirmed in randomized clinical trials, including taking them for the purpose of primary or secondary prevention of chronic diseases, such as cardiovascular disease, cancer, cognitive decline and effects on overall mortality.[197,198] The best thing you can do to get all the vitamins and minerals you need is to eat a healthy, balanced diet.

Dietary micronutrient deficiency is increasingly rare in developed countries, and people may not realize that by taking MVMs they might contribute to an excess vitamin and mineral intake, leading to toxicity. Doses higher than 500 mg/d of pyridoxine (vitamin B6), for example, have reported side effects of photosensitivity (higher sensitivity to the sun) and neurotoxicity,[199] and cases of pyridoxine-associated chronic sensory polyneuropathy in elderly patients.[200] Doses of 800–1200 mg/d of vitamin E can result in bleeding, and doses above 1200 mg/d have been reported to lead to diarrhea, weakness, blurred vision, and hormonal dysfunction.[201] Patients taking vitamin E supplementation following radiation therapy for head and neck cancer attracted national attention when there was an attributed increase in cancer recurrence in the first three-and-a-half years of follow-up[202] and increase in all-cause mortality.[203]

β-carotene supplements (vitamin A) have attracted widespread national attention because of an attributed significantly increased risk of lung cancer and increased mortality in male smokers,[204] an increased fracture risk,[205] and prostate cancer incidence[206] and mortality[207] in male alcohol users consuming a β-carotene supplement. High incidence of congenital abnormalities was reported in women who consumed large amounts of vitamin A supplements during pregnancy.[208] Minerals such as iron, often included in multivitamins, if consumed in excess alone or exacerbated by alcohol consumption could contribute to liver injury.[209,210]

To be on the safe side, you will not "miss the boat" or save money if you stay away from MVMs, unless you are pregnant, have confirmed nutritional deficiencies (such as vitamin B12 or folic acid) or have other risk factors that predispose you for them (a history of bariatric surgery, Crohn's disease, taking certain seizure or autoimmune disease medications). The upshot is, when you're considering a dietary supplement or multivitamin, start with taking foods that have an abundance of the supplement you intend to take instead.

Hoping for the safety of "natural" products, we may also underestimate the danger of interactions between supplements and conventional treatments. Dietary supplements could have an impact on surgery, anesthesia, and bloodwork interpretation. Use of supplements with blood-thinning medications, especially warfarin, can decrease their effect or increase risk of bleeding. The medicinal herb St John's wort (*Hypericum perforatum*) used for mood enhancement and depression, prominently interacts with HIV medications, contraceptives, immunosuppressants, antidepressants, and cancer drugs by changing the effects of these medications.[211]

Are you concerned about the safety of a supplement? Include all dietary supplements in your medication list with the name of manufacturer and the dose you take and treat them with the same caution as medications. Educate yourself about the length of treatment, doses, and interactions they can have with other medications. If you take any long-term medications, discuss with your physician the potential interactions before starting any supplement.

MISCONCEPTIONS ABOUT THE REGULATION OF DIETARY SUPPLEMENTS

Both patients and physicians seem to have widespread misconceptions about the regulation of dietary supplements. Supplements are regulated in the US by several federal agencies: the Food and Drug Administration (FDA) and the Federal Trade Commission (FTC); enforced by the State Attorneys General Offices (AGO) and Department of Justice (DOJ); and monitored (not regulated) by the Centers for Disease Control and Prevention (CDC).[212] The FDA regulates dietary supplements, but differently from other medications sold to consumers in the pharmacy. A manufacturer of a medication is required to document its effectiveness and safety before it can be brought to the market. In contrast, the FDA is not authorized to review dietary supplements for safety and effectiveness *before* they are marketed, leaving this responsibility to the manufacturers and distributors.

If the dietary supplement contains a *new* ingredient, manufacturers must notify the FDA about that ingredient prior to marketing it. However, the notification will only be reviewed by the FDA (not approved) and only for safety, not effectiveness. The requirements for safety of dietary supplements are much less stringent than for regular medications. No clinical trials are required for dietary supplements. Ingredients sold in the US before 15 October 1994 do not need safety evaluation by the FDA, as they are generally recognized as safe based on their historical use. The manufacturer must only notify the FDA for a new dietary ingredient not sold before 15 October 1994 and provide reasonable evidence that it is safe for human consumption.

Once a dietary supplement is on the market, the FDA tracks side effects reported by consumers, supplement companies and others. If the FDA finds a product to be unsafe, it can take legal action against the manufacturer or distributor and may issue a warning or require that the product be removed from the marketplace. However, the FDA says it can't test all products marketed as dietary supplements and they may contain potentially harmful hidden ingredients.[213] There is no requirement for demonstrating the efficacy of a dietary supplement for any health condition. Manufacturers of dietary supplements are not allowed to claim that the supplement can be used for treating or preventing any particular disease.

While companies are responsible for having evidence that their dietary supplements are safe, and that labels are truthful and not misleading, this is not always a reality. Rules for manufacturing and distributing dietary supplements are less strict than those for prescription or OTC drugs. What's on the label may not be what's in the product. Some dietary supplements can be harmful because of the tampering and contamination with detectable lead, mercury or arsenic, as well as undeclared pharmaceutical drugs.[214]

Manufacturers are required to produce supplements in accordance with Current Good Manufacturing Practices (CGMP), which is a registration program and set of standards enforced by the FDA. Adherence to the CGMP regulations assures the identity, strength, quality and purity of drug products by requiring that manufacturers of medications adequately control manufacturing operations.[215] Look for the CGMP stamp on the label of the dietary supplement you plan to use. That seal confirms that the manufacturer complies with all standards, procedures and documentation regarding its identity, strength, purity, and more. If a company is not complying with CGMP regulations, any drug it makes is considered "adulterated" under the law.[216] There are other quality stamps from third-party companies with unbiased assurance of quality criteria and who provide verification for dietary supplements, which you can look for on labels.

The National Sanitation Foundation (NSF) is an independent certification program that grants its seal of approval to products meeting purity standards in accordance with NSF/ANSI 173, an American National Standard that sets strict standards for the ingredients used in dietary supplements. NSF evaluates products for unacceptable levels of contaminants, such as heavy metals (for example, lead, arsenic), pesticides and herbicides, and confirms that their label accurately displays all ingredients, and that the product is compliant with CGMPs.[217]

Would you feel cheated if a claimed "natural" supplement had not one but two pharmaceuticals in it? Prescription drugs, including anticoagulants, antiseizure medications and drugs prescribed for erectile dysfunction were discovered in some dietary supplements. These powerful drugs, if taken uncontrolled, in high doses or in conjunction with other medications, can bring about devastating side effects. That's why you have to look for CGMP, NTF and USP stamps on the labels of dietary products.

The US Pharmacopeia (USP) is another independent quality

evaluation program that evaluates supplement and pharmaceutical drug quality. Products bearing a USP seal must conform to all USP standards, including:

- Identity: the supplement contains all ingredients indicated on the label.

- Potency: the potency of the product indicated on the label is accurately represented.

- Purity: the supplement is free of contaminants and unlabeled ingredients.

- Performance: the supplement dissolves, which allows the body to absorb the active ingredients.[218]

To maintain USP certification, manufacturers must undergo routine site and product inspections as well as random testing of off-the-shelf products displaying their seal.[219]

DISCUSSING DIETARY SUPPLEMENTS WITH CLINICIANS

Every dietary supplement's website recommends discussing supplements with your clinician, especially when you have chronic medical conditions, are taking prescription drugs or are preparing for surgery. This is what should be happening. The reality is slightly different.

A lot of patients believe that physicians don't have enough knowledge about nutritional supplements to provide substantive feedback.[220] Unfortunately, there is merit in that statement. According to researchers from Johns Hopkins University, who looked into physicians' knowledge of dietary supplements, of physicians from 15 Internal Medicine residency programs throughout the US, one-third were unaware that dietary supplements didn't require FDA approval or submission of safety and efficacy data before being marketed. Most physicians were unaware that serious adverse events should be reported.[221]

Most physicians have limited training in supplement use and have a limited knowledge in the regulation of them and side effects reporting, and therefore avoid discussing them with their patients.[222,223] In one study, which questioned 410 physicians about their conversation about supplements with their patients, more than 25 percent of physicians didn't feel comfortable handling clinical questions related to supplement use, and only 18 percent indicated they had a dependable source about supplement efficacy.[224]

In studies, while most clinicians agree that knowledge of complementary and alternative medicines (CAM) and conventional medicine is better than knowledge of prescription medicine alone, almost all felt that healthcare professionals need more education on CAM and that more research is necessary on the safety of CAM. What does this mean for patients? Until clinicians are trained in CAM and feel assured about its safety, scientific merit, and the regulations of recommending CAM safely, they will be reluctant to discuss or recommend CAM use.[225]

Fear "to cause harm" mixed with deep-rooted beliefs in evidence-based medicine alone have also made me cautious about dietary supplements. I pushed away my Siberian medical university upbringing notion of using centuries-long healing alternative medicine remedies to fit into the American doctor image. For years, I used the same strategy of looking for the information on the trusted NIH websites and giving it to my patients, encouraging them to make their own informed decisions. This has frequently brought on an embarrassing feeling of incompetency.

After being diagnosed with an illness that science doesn't have definite answers about, like many others I started looking for all available resources, including alternative medicine. I decided to get deep and real into the field of integrative medicine by joining the Andrew Weil Center for Integrative Medicine fellowship. Integrative medicine

neither rejects conventional medicine nor accepts alternative therapies uncritically and promotes patient and clinician partnership in
the healing process.[226] It was a pleasant surprise to see physicians of all
specialties among my fellowship colleagues, including surgery, oncology, pediatrics, neurology, rheumatology, cardiology, gastroenterology, and anesthesiology, from all over the world. We connected in
the desire to get the knowledge of healing interventions that didn't
fit into our daily conventional practices and therefore didn't reach
our patients, desperate in their need. We didn't learn CAM knowledge in medical school but were open-minded to join our patients in
their inquiry-driven search. If almost half of our patients used alternative medicine methods,[227] we felt inspired not only to "join the
boat," but to navigate it in the science-driven direction.

WHAT QUESTIONS SHOULD YOU ASK YOUR CLINICIAN BEFORE STARTING DIETARY SUPPLEMENTS?

Focus on safety, and not just the safety of the supplement. What
problem are you trying to fix? Is your fatigue actually a sign of chronic
illness or a side effect of another medication? Is your back pain a sign
of metastatic lytic lesions of unknown cancer, or do you need physical therapy? Are you trying to get a quick fix for a problem that needs
attention and additional work up that you are avoiding? What are
the chances that your illness progresses while you take the supplement? Supplements are not intended to treat an illness and should
not be taken instead of conventional treatments.

Will it be effective for the symptoms you're trying to deal with,
or will it interact with ongoing treatments, for example, cancer, seizure disorders, mental health illness, pregnancy, or other medications
prescribed or over the counter?

Learn and ask questions about the manufacturer, doses, side effects,
interactions, and a timeframe that is safe to take the supplement. Use

online resources[228] to identify the dietary supplement's safety profile-[229]and reliable manufacturers.[230]

Be particularly cautious with combined supplements that have multiple ingredients. Bring them to your visit with your clinician. Some supplements can exacerbate your existing medical conditions. For example, caffeine in pre-workout supplements will increase your blood pressure and may be the reason for your palpitations. Keep in mind that dietary supplements may contain ingredients not listed on the label and might need to be taken for a long period of time to achieve the promised effect, which also might not be confirmed in reliable clinical trials.

Do not assume that every clinician has comprehensive knowledge of dietary supplements, regulations, manufacturers, and adverse effects. Be bold and ask about their expertise in that area. Ask your clinician if they feel comfortable giving you advice about supplements. Alternatively, seek advice from an Integrative Medicine practitioner, who, in addition to medical knowledge, has graduated from an Integrative Medicine fellowship or is board-certified in Integrative Medicine.

CHECK YOUR HEALTHCARE INVENTORY:

If you take dietary supplements:

1. Check whether they have stamps of "quality control" from the FDA and/or independent manufacturers: CGMP, USP, NSF. If they don't, consider a supplement that does.

2. Check the safety profile of all your supplements.

3. Include all of them in your medication list to consult with your clinicians about whether they are effective for your medical problems and will not interact with other medications you take, either prescribed or over the counter.

CHAPTER 18

TO ERR IS HUMAN

At times of uncertainty, errors are inevitable. But not all errors are created equally. Diagnostic error is a leading type of all medical errors because making complex decisions under uncertainty is hard, even for experts. Daniel Kahneman PhD, an Israeli-born psychologist, together with Amos Tversky PhD, who unexpectedly died before the award nomination, was awarded the Nobel Memorial Prize in Economics for their groundbreaking work in the areas of decision-making under uncertainty.

Their experiments showed that human brains utilize two types of decision-making. One is unconscious, fast and intuitive, whereas the other is systematic, analytical, effort intensive, and much slower. Complex decision-making requires a combination of both types of thinking.[231] Human brains have limits of cognitive capacity and develop a multitude of frameworks or shortcuts to help us organize, sort, and use information.[232] Decision-making shortcuts are known as heuristics, a simple decision strategy that ignores part of the available information and focuses on the few more familiar predictors.[233] Both patients and doctors are susceptible to those heuristics.

To relatively healthy patients, or patients with controlled medical problems, death seems remote. It's much more comforting to concentrate on the feeling of being in control of current health conditions than face "new risks" of fatal illness, which seem too remote to consider.[234] *Attention judgment* heuristics are common for patients with chronic medical conditions or physicians involved in their care. Their focus on selective, specific information related to chronic illness prevents them from considering alternative diseases, potentially missing early stages of other illnesses, including cancer.[235] Carlos, for example, concentrated on control of his diabetes, high blood pressure and cholesterol and did not even consider the possibility of colon cancer while having symptoms of frequent stooling.

The *framing effect* is more common than we think. "My husband had two glasses of Scotch that evening. We argued about his alcohol intake. I thought he was drunk and didn't pay attention when his speech got slurred," said the wife of one of my patients who'd had a stroke, and which wasn't acknowledged until half of his body was paralyzed. She felt terrible. "I even got mad, telling him, 'You see what alcohol does to you, the doctor said you shouldn't be drinking because of your blood pressure!' I left him alone, instead of rushing him to the hospital…" She simply relied on her previous impression of her husband as a "drinker;" her brain used the shortcut of the framing effect because of how we're influenced by the way information is presented.

The probability of cancer in young patients seems low for patients and doctors, in comparison with the probability of other causes of symptoms more common for young people. Yet young adults are 58 percent more likely to be diagnosed with late-stage colorectal cancer than older people, showing a strong bias of the age framing effect.[236]

Premature closure is a type of cognitive error in which we, both patients and physicians, fail to explore reasonable alternatives after an initial diagnosis is made, leading to delayed diagnosis and misdiagnosis. An example was Matt and Kristen.

"You look stunning!" said Matt, looking at his bride. There she stood in a rose-white embroidered wedding dress, happily smiling, satisfied with her 15lb weight loss to fit into her mother's wedding dress, which had been beautifully restored. Kristen was in college when she'd met Matt, an engineer who'd just transferred to Charleston to start his new managerial role. They had a beautiful southern wedding, surrounded by 200 family and friends under the large oaks of Boone Hall Plantation. Storytelling from the Gullah culture sent uplifting spiritual messages of love and understanding and how overcoming the hardships of the past can lead to a better place today. Little did Kristen know that she would need that strength soon after.

Kristen was 27 years old when she started seeking help for the cramps in her abdomen. Initially, she thought the cramps were from the stress of planning the wedding. She'd wanted to fit into her wedding dress, but the weight loss didn't stop after the wedding. Her primary care doctor ordered laboratory tests. All came back normal. She was advised to change her diet, visit her gynecologist, and start new birth control pills. She changed doctors. She was referred to the gastroenterologist, but her endoscopic studies were also normal, and she was told that she had irritable bowel syndrome. Insurance didn't approve a CT of her abdomen. Only after a repeated pelvic ultrasound showed fluid in her abdomen did a CT of the abdomen and pelvis show not only fluid but liver metastasis. The melanoma was advanced by the time the diagnosis was established.

Going back to Carlos, he interpreted his frequent bowel movements as the result of a high-fiber diet. This quick judgment and his following actions were promptly available in his memory. Carlos had changed his diet to treat his diabetes and cholesterol and had succeeded. He wanted to lose weight and thought that frequent bowel movements would help him to achieve his goal. In his mind, a high-fiber diet was connected to his new symptom in a positive way. This brain shortcut is called an availability heuristic, based on the most available information in our long-term memory.

Heuristics take place when we must think quickly at a time of uncertainty. Doctors learn about the powers and pitfalls of heuristics shortcuts in school, and how they may help to save lives, but can also lead to diagnostic errors. Patients can be guided by heuristics under emotional pressure of feelings without being aware of the brain tricks influencing their judgment and actions.

Bill Stags was taking the "purple pill," or omeprazole, over the counter to reduce symptoms of heartburn that had started three weeks prior. Omeprazole belongs to the group of proton pump inhibitors (PPIs), which 15 million Americans regularly use every year. One day, Bill's "heartburn" brought on dizziness that he hadn't experienced before. Suddenly, he wasn't able to walk and lost consciousness.

An ambulance arrived quickly, which saved his life. It took almost six hours for cardiovascular surgeons to repair his dissecting aortic aneurysm. Dissection of the aorta is a critical condition that has a mortality rate of 60 percent. When a tear occurs in the inner layer of the largest artery, blood passes through the tear, spreading into the inner and middle layers of the aorta, causing dissection. People may experience back pain or stomach pain, and this may take some time. If the blood penetrates to outside the aortic wall, aortic dissection is often deadly. When an aortic dissection is detected early and treated, the chances of survival greatly improve. Did Bill know about other reasons behind the burning feeling in his chest? When he experienced symptoms of chest pain, his brain made a shortcut to indigestion and the "purple pill" he'd heard about many times and seen in TV commercials.

Diagnostic error is a nightmare for patients and physicians. Patients lose trust in healthcare and clinicians in general. Physicians scrutinize their cognitive processes. The fear of diagnostic error can change a physician's behavior, such as ordering more tests and therefore making healthcare more expensive than it should be. Multiple patient safety practices have been established in healthcare to make it safer: clinical decision support, result notification systems, education and training, and peer-reviewed procedures.

Do they always work? Systems can malfunction for many reasons. This is where patients can and should step in—by taking a greater role in your own healthcare, being informed, following your own progress, looking for available resources, asking questions, seeking a second opinion, closing the loop between your symptoms, diagnoses, and treatments, and sharing your thoughts in the medical decision-making process.

Medical errors are frightening for patients and doctors. I have been on both sides of medical errors: as a patient and a doctor.

My mother wasn't just an experienced surgeon. She was a surgeon in Siberia, who as skillfully as she operated on the heart did so on the abdomen. She had questioned her diagnosis of stomach flu in her only child and asked for advice from her superior professor, who was a wise, well-respected expert, and who'd never had children but knew the ethical rule: do not treat your own family. There was no CT scanner at that time, just the feel and touch of an expert physician who made a diagnosis.

I remember the room was white and chilling cold. Forget about warm blankets, which are given to patients even for small procedures in US hospitals. I remember the brightness of the large operating room light focused on the opening in the surgical drape, exposing the right side of my belly. I'd seen this ritual of covering patients with white drapes many times while watching my mother performing surgeries from the top benches of the OR. Today, it was my chubby and tall 14-year-old teenager-self lying on the cold operating table looking at the bright light of the lamps. I felt pain, a deep pulling on my guts. Since then, I've had doubts about local anesthesia used for abdominal surgeries. Thank God for the invention of epidural anesthesia, and, at that time, the magical effect of medication making people forget about everything that happened during surgery was missing. I didn't have either. I was there, remembering the light and pain of my own appendectomy.

She is so slow, I was thinking. *If she moves her hands as slowly as she walks, I will die here from pain.* The needle sticks were sharply noted in my pain journey, but it was a deep, heavy, crashing pain when I started hearing the sound of sweat drops reach the marble floor of the OR. One drop. Two drops.

When my tiny pale appendix was examined by a pathologist, the verdict was that I didn't have appendicitis. My mother was right, and the expert surgeon professor was wrong. There had been no need for me to lie down on that cold, hard operating table and let the slow fingers pull my guts out. When my mother's resident checked out my wound the next day, I heard a sound that wasn't a sign of admiring technical skill. The size of the new scar was triple the size that beginner surgeons make to remove the appendix. It was a technical inconvenience detail on top of diagnostic error that prevented me from wearing a bikini for the rest of my life. I was silent and even tried to smile when I saw my mother's red eyes full of tears. We never talked about it. We make mistakes. Doctors make mistakes.

DEFENSIVE MEDICINE

On 29 November 1999, the Institute of Medicine (IOM) released a report starting with poet Alexander Pope's famous words: *To Err is Human*, but ending with, "Building a Safer Health System by recognizing the aim of healthcare quality for the benefits of patients' safety."[237] The popular proverbial phrase "To err is human" in its original form has a different ending: "To err is human; to forgive, divine."[238]

The landmark report of the IOM suggested that human errors are inevitable. Doctors are human. Yet when doctors make mistakes, even when they suffer with and without a patient, they lose their licenses and credibility in front of insurance companies to practice the only field they know, the only passion they have. They also face a judge for their unintentional errors in the same rooms where murderers and rapists plead guilty for their crimes. Even after doctors pay for the errors with the cost of their homes and savings, they continue to suffer for unintentionally hurting someone else because the first thought of the doctor's pledge enters our hearts: "Do no harm." You can only take it with a hammer or knife from those hearts.

The fear of unintentionally hurting someone as well as a desire to reduce exposure to damage claims of malpractice leads many to practice *defensive medicine*. A punitive approach to error in hospitals encourages the culture of not exposing the error, instead of learning from it.

I know what you're thinking—what would you say if your loved one was hurt by someone's human error? Well, let me tell you about my own error.

Girls love to be cheerleaders. Being at the center of the football field, in pretty uniforms, flying up to the sky, being caught by the supportive hands of your teammates. If everything goes right. Who doesn't want that? What if it doesn't go right? Cheerleading is the most dangerous female sport when we look at the number of catastrophic injuries. High-school cheerleading accounted for 65.2 percent of all high-school female catastrophic sports injuries in 2009.[239] My daughter dreamed about cheerleading and practiced all kinds of stunts on the grass of our backyard. She was flawless. She practiced with the notion that if she knew what she was doing, injury wouldn't happen. That's how we think. But it will happen if your teammate next to you doesn't do her part. Another human error.

Under the heavier weight of her teammate, my little girl's leg stumbled. She fell and her teammate landed on top of her. She couldn't step on the leg, which immediately swelled. We used the RICE principle of rest, ice, compression, and elevation as a first aid for all injuries. But two weeks of the RICE principle didn't bring the expected relief. "Why are you limping?" I asked my daughter who, like an injured bird, was hopping in front of me one evening when we were on our way out to eat. Sadly, this famous question became a lifelong reminder of my own medical error. I made an error not as a doctor, but, more importantly, I made this error as her mother. Which one is worse?

Next day, my sports medicine colleague, who I asked to look at my daughter's leg, said, in an understanding way, "This is loosey-goosey," meaning signs of knee instability. I'd missed the diagnosis of a complicated ACL and meniscal injury thinking it was a mild ligament sprain. "Why are you still limping?" The words haunted me.

After ACL repair surgery, and eight weeks of intense physical therapy, my athletic child couldn't run. What kind of mother was I? Didn't I know about the dangers of cheerleading as a sport? I saw patients with ligament sprains every day, many times a day. What kind of doctor was I? Why would I make this mistake on my daughter?

My yoga instructor, Sarah, told me once when I tried to practice a headstand in my late forties, "Pain is your teacher. You feel pain, stop, listen, still push a little. If the pain gets worse, go back and stay there." It was a wisdom that I have practiced since. I took my daughter to my yoga instructor. She started taking yoga classes with a bunch of other people, driven to yoga for peace of mind, strength, and the simple principle "do what you can do in the moment." It healed her spirit and her knee. She felt pain, pushed a little further and there was no pain. She pushed through and was running four weeks later. Yoga also healed me from the pain of my error.

The ethical code "Do not treat family members" is based on the competing personal and professional expectations. Our profession emphasizes detached objectivity and scientific inquiry, while the illness of a loved one provokes an emotional involvement that can cloud critical thinking and reasonableness. Despite all known rules, physicians feel compelled in favor of involvement. I start my lecture about medical errors with my own mistakes.

Robin Robins, an ABC anchor, once said, "Make a message out of your mess." In clinical practice, human errors are generally underreported. As a result of this, we lose the chance to know about the causes and consequences of medical errors. Some estimates indicate that the practice of defensive medicine costs $46 billion annually in the United States.[240] But it is necessary to face the situation and learn from it to prevent future errors.

When my kids ask me what to do with a headache, cough or pain, I take a deep breath and say, "Why are you limping?" reminding them about my motherly biased tendency to make mistakes and inviting them into the mutual discussion about what's happening and what we should do about it. I listen to my patients' stories and their opinions before I make my own judgment call, in spite of my knee-jerk reaction to make a diagnosis right away. *Fix it*, keeps running through my mind. *Slow down my fast and furious mind. Do my patients want it to be fixed? How do my patients want it to be fixed? Will treatment be worse than a disease?*

As much as every healthcare professional wants and intends to provide safe care, medical errors could happen at any point of medical care. Patients can suffer from mistaken identifiers and erroneous medical records to improper transfusions, misdiagnosis, under and overtreatment, surgical injuries and wrong-site surgery, suicides, restraint-related injuries or in hospital falls, infections, pressure ulcers, and communication between providers and the patient and a family.[241]

Medication errors are among those where patients, if involved in their own care, can make a big difference. Medication error is a failure in the treatment process that leads to, or has the potential to lead to, harm to the patient.[242] Medication errors are the cause of one in every 131 outpatient and one in every 854 inpatient deaths.[243] Complexities of pharmacology, healthcare delivery and miscommunication in transitions are the major contributors to medication errors. They can be the result of either the medications themselves, healthcare professionals or patient actions. Medication errors might occur during each of the three steps involving medication use: prescribing, dispensing and while taking medications.

I remember Elizabeth Cornwell, a 62-year-old administrative assistant who had a talent for organization. She had a precise schedule for all her events, tasks, appointments, and records, even after she retired after 30 years in a law office. Being the eldest child in a family of six children, she had learned early that order will cut out a lot of unnecessary work and saves time. Her appointments were timely placed in her calendar and an alarm on her phone notified her when it was time for medications. She had hypothyroidism and took daily levothyroxine to supplement her thyroid function, always at the same time. Every six months she got a blood test to check the level of her thyroid hormone, to make sure her supplementation dose met her body's needs. She felt good about herself that she was able to fix another problem by organizing her life.

After the last blood draw, a nurse from the clinic called her with the lab results and explained that the level of thyroid hormone was low, and the dose of levothyroxine had to be increased. The new dose of levothyroxine was sent to her pharmacy. Elizabeth purchased the new dose and started taking it in addition to the old levothyroxine dose, thinking that was the difference that was needed to supplement her low blood level of thyroid hormone.

Two weeks later, she noticed her heart pounding, almost as if she had been running a mile. She attributed it to higher stress and decided not to watch the news that night. Eventually, her heartbeat became so fast she couldn't catch her breath. In the ED she was told she had irregular heartbeats due to chaotic electrical signals from her heart, a condition called atrial fibrillation. When heartbeats happen that fast and irregularly, it can lead to blood clots, stroke, heart failure and other heart-related complications. Elizabeth's heart was beating 190 beats per minute, triggered by the high dose of levothyroxine. She was started on medication to decrease her heartrate. When she let her doctors in the hospital know that the dose had changed two weeks before, it became clear that medical error had occurred. Elizabeth had taken the old and the new doses of levothyroxine together, instead of switching from the old dose to the new dose. Elizabeth suffered from the medication error.

ERRORS OF OMISSION

If you're discharged from hospital and one of the medications you've previously taken isn't on the discharge list, should you take it or not? You don't remember talking to the doctor in the hospital about this medication, but you don't want the hassle of reaching out to your hospital team. Instead, you start taking your previous old medication, ignoring the fact that you may have potential interactions with newly prescribed drugs. This is an *error of omission*.

To avoid this type of error, patients are advised to provide an accurate list of medications. Clinicians should reconcile it during each healthcare encounter in the primary care setting, specialist office or hospital. Reconciliation helps to identify medications that must be stopped and new medications that must be started. However, there are two issues with this well-designed process: one, only every third (27.9 percent) patient could list their discharge medications, and even fewer could state their intended use;[244] and two, despite medication reconciliation being initially mandated 15 years ago as a universal process for every inpatient or outpatient encounter, more than 40 percent of medication errors are believed to result from inadequate reconciliation in handoffs during admission, transfer and discharge of patients. Of these errors, about 20 percent are believed to result in harm.[245,246]

While physicians try to fix reconciliation issues, patients' awareness of their long-term medications can help with over half of potential medical errors. We are accustomed to having a passport while traveling from one country to another; we don't question its necessity. I wish we accepted this mandate for medication lists too; it would save more lives than our compliance with passports. *Your medication list is your medical passport, so give it the attention it deserves.*

ERRORS OF COMMISSION

When a clinician prescribes a medication to which a patient has an allergy—because allergies to medications weren't verified during the visit, or when a patient takes the wrong dose of a medication—these are *errors of commission.*

In patients with decreased kidney function, as a result of diabetes, high blood pressure or chronic renal disease, doses of many medications have to be adjusted individually based on the laboratory testing.[247] When you ask a new physician to refill medications, they might not be aware of your renal function compromise and prescribe a dose that is too high, leading to medication error. Having your most recent laboratory results available could help to prevent this.

The challenges in interoperability of health records makes it virtually impossible to know current medication lists, unless patients verify them. A small blue pill and a bigger pink pill is an additional mystery the medical team has to solve by calling pharmacies, unless patients again bring clarity by bringing their medications to the visit. Yes, medical professionals accept their detective role and can figure it out, but it can take time from your visit and there is also the potential for error.

You might think, *Pharmacies dispense medications, so they know what medications I should take.* Another misconception! Pharmacies know what medications have been prescribed, but they aren't informed about what medications have been discontinued.

Most people assume that when they establish care with a new doctor or visit a specialist and inform them about their medications, this doctor critically assesses their medications. Some doctors are under the assumption that the medication list was previously reconciled, and all medications are necessary for treatment of other medical problems. Time restriction is also a barrier for questions, such as, is this medication the best option for my treatment? Could this medication be responsible for symptoms I'm currently dealing with?

Michael Werner had been seeing a pulmonologist and underwent extensive workup because of his dry cough, which had been bothering him for the last 12 months. He had pulmonary function tests, a chest x-ray and even chest CT, which all returned without explanation of his chronic cough. The pulmonologist referred Michael to a gastroenterologist to evaluate potential reasons for his persistent cough. Michael underwent upper endoscopy and was found to have mild symptoms of GERD and started to take omeprazole to treat it.

After three months of treatment, the cough continued, and the gastroenterologist referred him to a cardiologist, who also performed a series of even more expensive tests that, as you may guess, didn't find the reasons for the cough. Michael was advised to establish with a primary care physician for "cancer screenings." When he showed up in our clinic, you could see his lack of trust and frustration. "I don't like doctors," was the first thing that came out of his mouth. He brought a stack of documents with his extensive workup from three specialists to avoid duplication of expensive procedures.

Michael Werner had a long history of hypertension, which was well controlled with a small dose of ramipril, which he'd been taking for ten years. Ramipril belongs to the group of powerful antihypertensive drugs called angiotensin-converting enzyme (ACE) inhibitors. ACE inhibitors block angiotensin-converting enzyme, which tightens blood vessels. Blocking this chemical makes blood vessels more relaxed and brings blood pressure down. ACE inhibitors are not expensive and are effective for controlling blood pressure, preventing stroke and heart attacks. But ACE inhibitors, including ramipril, frequently cause a mild, annoying dry cough. Neither Michael nor other physicians suspected the side effect because Michael had taken it for ten years and the cough had started 12 months ago. Three weeks after Michael stopped ramipril, his cough was gone.

Most physicians I spoke to about this book cautioned me not to write about medical errors or defensive behaviors. Are there expectations that doctors are some type of superhero equipped with the magic touch or a powerful genie in a bottle? Or is it some type of stoicism doctors should portray or express in order to be trusted, or is it a culture of individual blame that prevents doctors and patients from honestly talking about risks of tests and treatments?

A common assumption in the blame culture, which is in line with the legal system, is that people make mistakes because they don't pay enough attention to the tasks, or they do things they're not adequately skilled for. As a result, blame is directed toward people who actually took courage and shared their knowledge and skills. The risk of losing face and the fear of legal disputes are powerful incentives for doctors to hide errors and engage in defensive behaviors. There is another option, where instead of looking for a person to blame and punish, successful health organizations promote the principle of shared decision-making and involve patients in collaborative communication.

We are all human: doctors and patients. We learn and keep learning from our own and others' mistakes. We need our colleagues and teammates to remind us about things we may forget, miss or misunderstand. It's impossible to do this alone. We need our patients' watchful eye and commonsense judgments, questions, reminders, and opinions at every step of medical care. Bring them on!

CHECK YOUR HEALTHCARE INVENTORY:

1. Do you have different doctors involved in your care? Keep track of changes of treatment and medications by looking at the patient portal or getting a printed summary of your visit with your medication list.

2. When tests are ordered, don't assume that if you do not get a notification about the results that they are normal. Check the results, ask questions about their meaning, whether tests need to be repeated and when.

CHAPTER 19

A "GOOD" DOCTOR

*"Medicine is only for those who
cannot imagine doing anything else."*

Luanda Grazette, Cardiologist

Everyone wants to be treated by a *good* doctor, but what makes a *good* doctor? We search through doctors' biographies online trying to find the qualities that make a "good" doctor. Does it matter why people become doctors, or what medical school and residency they graduated from? Are degrees in Doctors of Osteopathy (DO) and Medical Doctors (MD) the same? Can doctors from foreign medical schools be trusted the same as US graduates? Are women doctors more caring than men? Does experience matter? How do you find the one whose knowledge and expertise you can trust?

In comparison with young people who aren't sure about their future aspirations, decisions about being a doctor are often made early in life. A quarter of clinicians had decided that they would be applying for medical school even before attending high school.[248] An interest in people, the role of doctors in society and a desire to serve society have been named as the main motives for wanting to study medicine by the majority of doctors.[249,250] Even more, an "interest in people" continues to be a driving force for people to stay in this demanding profession for at least 20 years and has predicted future physicians' satisfaction with their jobs.[251] The intention to have a "prestigious profession" was also ranked close, by three out of five doctors. The value of joy in their profession with a "wide range of professional opportunities" overpowered a "good salary."[252] Medicine is the most inherited elite career. Doctors' children are 24 times more likely to enter the field of medicine than their peers.[253] Is it intergenerational transfers of passion that drive children to follow their parents' footsteps, or stories of being someone's hero by saving lives, or an infectious feeling of joy after altruistic acts? Is it a prepared path to success nurtured by a doctor parent? Influence by parents and the perceived respect in society ranked high in studies of motivations to becoming a doctor.[254]

I didn't know any of those statistics when, at age 17, I made my choice from three career aspirations: dancer, spy or doctor. In Russia, kids can bypass college and enter six years of education at a medical school right after high school. What I did not know then was that being a doctor would put all my dreams together: doctors have to think like detectives, figuring out clues to make a diagnosis; they accept the risks between life and death, and they have to do a communication dance with patients. At the Family Medicine graduation party at Duke University, my mentor, a great doctor and teacher, Dr. Andy Bonin, gave me a black and white feather boa as a graduation gift. "Maria practices medicine like dancing tango. She pivots and makes brisk, calculated, gracious and precise steps." He didn't know then that he'd given me the best compliment as a dancer I had ever received.

I did not know then that doctors were also "detectives." I loved puzzles, taking risks and listening to stories, but wasn't adventurous or determined enough to become a spy. Medicine was close and familiar for a girl who'd grown up in a house always full of medical students, residents and my mother's doctor colleagues. Listening to their excitement at new discoveries and wonders, medicine seemed fun and promised a lot of puzzles that needed to be solved and stories to listen to.

HIGH CALLING

There is usually a role-model, parent, family friend or even a doctor who influences young people to get into the "high-calling" medical profession. Medical students frequently describe a powerful event or illness with a successful cure that triggers feelings of compassion to humankind, and which drives young people into medicine. For me it was medical failure, or to be precise, my mother's failure to recognize the early signs of her own breast cancer. Being too busily involved in her patients' medical cures, she missed her own illness. After decades of practicing medicine, I learned what good doctors do: they focus on others, they perpetually sacrifice and, surprisingly, enjoy doing it.

It's traditional to think of doctors as superhumans, attributable to a high-calling profession. But being seen as Superman or Wonder Woman is only enjoyable in the movies. Doctors' initial dreams of helping people become buried in myriad clerical tasks necessary for meeting health system requirements, long work hours, sleep deprivation with overnight calls, and high levels of stress under the pressure of personal responsibility for human lives. Starting from medical school, doctors experience depression, burnout, and mental illness at a higher rate than the general population, with mental health deteriorating over the course of training and later in practice.[255]

Every one or two years, while renewing a medical license or hospital privileges, physicians must answer an intrusive question: do you or did you have a mental illness? If mental illness is disclosed during the license application or renewal, it will most likely be followed by multiple medical assessments and a demand for access to all of the applicant's mental health records from psychiatrists, therapists and hospitals, and eventual legal consequences. Physicians fear that dis-closure of depression or anxiety in a licensure application might result in accusation by the medical board that they have filed a false application in the past. Concerns about lack of confidentiality, a negative impact on career, and stigma have prevented close to two-thirds of physicians from seeking help.

REVIEW YOUR EXPECTATIONS

It's hard to define a good doctor. Most professionals are judged by the end results. Lawyers: you won the lawsuit; you got your property or desired divorce. Contractors: your house is built. Services: your home is clean, internet works, roof doesn't leak. Patients' expectations of doctors are to be cured from illness, which, a lot of the time, is simply not possible. Cure is not a frequent outcome of many chronic illnesses, especially without patients' own efforts. Even by giving the correct advice to take a pill, there is a patient-dependent action component that might fail.

We have high expectations for doctors. Why not? By trusting doctors with our health, we presume that all doctors are knowledge-able, experienced, and trustworthy. Is this true? We also generalize expectations of the profession and apply them to individual people. As a result, patients view the entire person through this perfect label. What's wrong with this assumption that all doctors are great? What are your expectations for doctors?

Doctors are human beings, and as such they are not perfect. They have weaknesses, flaws, and imperfections. They get sick, divorced, and sometimes make the wrong financial decisions. As much as they try to follow the standards of the profession, they may never meet your expectations. When doctors don't look, listen or, God forbid, don't act as patients anticipate, those high expectations may be quickly crushed.

A doctor might be acting in your best interest and following guidelines by not prescribing unnecessary treatments, such as antibiotics for a common cold, opiates for pain that could be treated with simple Tylenol, or not ordering an expensive MRI for uncomplicated back pain. Instead of writing a quick prescription, doctors may spend longer convincing you that "do no harm" is the best option. They might act this way, despite knowing that you might consider them incompetent, heartless or inattentive or even write a bad review on social media about them. The old term of the "art of medicine" circulates in our minds despite physicians' intentions to practice scientific, evidence-based medicine.

Physicians are involved in the most regulated profession. Throughout their careers, doctors confirm and validate their ability to practice medicine over and over by renewing medical licenses, taking the required medical boards' continuous education, asking peers for references, and even reporting the status of their mental health to maintain their licenses to prove that they continue to be trustworthy and knowledgeable enough to take care of their patients. Powered by emotions and a deep intent to "do no harm," doctors sometimes feel compromised, torn by the obligations to follow protocols and guidelines.

HONESTY

Medicine has many gray areas with layers of uncertainty. When we discuss the risks of a procedure that could relieve someone's suffering, the potential complications, which are true, might be described as more frightening than the current suffering, and the patient will reject the procedure itself. If we undermine the potential complications, would that be incomplete disclosure and lying? Some patients prefer not to be told of a serious diagnosis but would rather a family member be informed instead. Or family members let the doctor know that the patient doesn't want to know. Withholding the truth is still common in some cultures, including my own.

Raisa Ivanova's family was protective of her when her chronic headache diagnosis changed to glioblastoma—terminal brain cancer. Episodes of dizziness were followed by memory loss. Her anxiety rose to the highest level. She didn't understand why this was happening, why multiple doctors visited, and why the treatments didn't lead to improvement. Her husband, who'd been her health power of attorney, begged me not to tell Raisa that the illness was terminal, and she might have just a few months left to live. They counted on my understanding of our Russian culture, which "spares" their loved one from the negative impact of an overbearing terminal diagnosis for as long as possible. Being torn between my obligations to my patient to tell the truth and my cultural beliefs did not let me sleep at night and were probably visible in my eyes during the visits.

"The pain of not being with my mother for her last years of life still follows me four decades later," I shared my personal painful experience with Raisa's husband, when he brought weak Raisa for a visit. "I wasn't given the chance to cherish the last moments with someone I loved the most." It's common in Russian culture to withhold the truth "to protect" loved ones. I found out about my mother's breast cancer two weeks before her death. For three years I had been intentionally sent away by my parents for different reasons to be "spared" the pain of knowing about her struggles through mastectomy, radiation, and her imminent death.

When Grigory, Raisa's husband, who by that time was legally making decisions about his wife's health, finally allowed me to share the diagnosis with Raisa, she said quietly, "I know. I've known for a while that I won't recover from this, whatever it is."

For a good doctor, even expertise is not enough. There are many jokes involving a priest, a doctor, and an attorney, which stresses the special value of professional expertise bound with personal relationships. These relationships have non-disclosure and lack-of-judgment prerequisites mixed in with patient vulnerability and trust.

DOES EXPERTISE MATTER?

The role of expertise in any field doesn't need defending. Clinical expertise consists of the ability to make the right decisions or clinical judgment and medical knowledge. What is more important, knowledge or judgment? Younger doctors are technically savvy, have social media communication skills and presence. They are knowledgeable about the latest medical advances. Would you be concerned about their clinical judgment because of fewer patients seen, fewer right decisions made, fewer errors that have happened, limited procedures and surgeries done? We still don't know how lapses of clinical judgment versus a lack of knowledge affect patient outcomes.

Doctors who are more confident in their physical exam findings order fewer tests. Primary care doctors with more experience seek less consultant advice, providing more affordable care.[256]

Dr. Niteesh K. Choudhry, with his colleagues from Harvard University, evaluated the relationship between quality of patient care, physicians' age and years in practice using a sample of more than 33,000 physicians. They concluded that while "practice makes perfect" in some situations, physicians' knowledge and performance may decline with the passage of time. They wrote, "physicians who have been in practice for more years and older physicians possess less factual knowledge, are less likely to adhere to appropriate standards of care, and may also have poorer patient outcomes. Medical advances occur frequently, and the explicit knowledge that physicians possess may easily become out of date as an explanation of late-career clinicians' reduced clinical knowledge, less adherence to treatment guidelines, and lower scores on quality measures for diagnosis, screening, and prevention."[257.]

As soon as this study was published, questions were raised about its methodologic quality, questioning its outcomes. What are the problems with older physicians' care? Physicians' "knowledge repositories" created during training may not be as technologically advanced as those of recent graduates. Older physicians may be less receptive to new standards of care and current guidelines, but they compensate through clinical judgment and sometimes valuing commonsense. Many experienced physicians have witnessed the rise and fall of guidelines and expert opinions and are quite skeptical of the measures of quality chosen for them.

Analysis of hospitalizations by 18,854 hospitalist physicians with a median physician age of 41 years, showed there was no association between a physician's age and 30-day patient mortality in care provided by physicians older than 60 years old with high-volume practices; however, higher patient mortality was observed with care provided by older physicians with low-volume practices.[258] Older doctors may lose on the knowledge scale to physicians straight out of residency, but the most important knowledge we get from residency is not the pieces of knowledge but how to think through the facts, how to judge them, how to apply them to real patients and how to make decisions.

With information easily available to all of us, there is no doubt that the problem of new knowledge can be fixed more easily than the problem of lack of clinical judgment. As patients, we have to exercise our own judgment about what we value the most: experience versus modern knowledge, giving preference to the balance between the two.

DOES GENDER MATTER?

When people choose a doctor of a certain gender, they are guided by their own perceptions. However, in clinical studies, when asked to choose physician experience, bedside manner, competency or gender, gender was ranked as the last selection.[259] Medicine is traditionally a male-dominated field with male doctors still outnumbering female doctors by almost half (64 percent to 36 percent), but this trend is changing.[260,261] Women doctors dominate in fields of obstetrics and gynecology, pediatrics, dermatology, allergy and immunology, genetics, and palliative care.

There are known gender differences in practicing medicine. Female physicians may be more likely to adhere to clinical guidelines,[262,263] provide preventive care more often,[264,265,266] use more patient-centered communication,[267] perform as well or better on standardized examinations,[268] and provide more psychosocial counseling to their patients than do their male peers.[269]

How about patient outcomes? Yusuke Tsugawa, with colleagues from Harvard T.H. Chan School of Public Health, analyzed outcomes of a random sample of 621,412 men and 961,616 women 65 years or older hospitalized with a medical condition and treated by general internists. They concluded that, "Elderly hospitalized patients treated by female internists have lower mortality and readmissions compared with those cared for by male internists."

Does this mean that, generally, women are better primary care doctors? I don't think so. Women's nurturing trend and communication styles help to win this gender race in doctoring. However, this couldn't and shouldn't be generalizable to surgical conditions, or patients treated by physicians of other specialties, or to outpatient care.[270] Individual level of comfort while being treated is different. In my experience, patients, for their own reasons, give preference to either a male or female physician, going "with your gut."

DOES MEDICAL SCHOOL MATTER?

The short answer is no. Having a highly ranked medical school in their professional background gives new physicians better opportunities for postgraduate training in the specialty of choice. But when it comes to patients, it does not matter. Most patients don't even know what school their doctors attended. Every fourth doctor in the US is an international medical graduate (IMG),[271] meaning that they graduated from non-US medical schools. I am one of them. On 16 June 1992, I came to the US with two kids, two bags and a big dream, as did thousands of immigrants.

To determine whether patient outcomes and cost of care differ between general internists who've graduated from a medical school outside the US and those who've graduated from a US medical school, Dr. Yusuke Tsugawa, with his colleagues from Harvard University, analyzed mortality rates of a random sample of 1,215,490 admissions to hospital treated by 44,227 general internists, 44 percent of them IMGs. They found that patients treated by the international graduates had a lower 30-day mortality rate than those treated by the US graduates. There were no differences in the readmission rates and a slightly higher spending for the international graduates. These differences persisted across a broad range of clinical conditions. International graduates who are successful in the US matching process might represent some of the best physicians in their country of origin because matching into the US residency is much more competitive for IMGs than for US graduates.

Many international graduates currently practicing in the US, including myself, likely underwent residency training twice—once in their home country and once in the US—and therefore have more experience and knowledge. As international graduates, we experience a loss of our profession when leaving our countries and are more concerned about potential professional failure, so perhaps we are more engaged in continuous training and updating our skills and knowledge. We know how painful the loss of profession can be.

DO WHAT WE PREACH

Physicians teach people to be healthy as part of their job. Do they follow their own advice? Most of the time they do.

As a group, physicians have healthier lifestyles and lower mortality rates than the general public. Male physicians win in the area of focusing on wellness, physical and spiritual health in comparison with women. Physicians tend to have good health habits compared with the general population. Physicians' personal wellness has an influence on how they promote preventive practices to their patients. Physicians who follow wellness principles in their own lives have a positive impact on the health practices of their patients, such as mammography, colorectal cancer screening and vaccinations.[272] This is proven on the lifestyle habits of exercise, smoking and making healthy food choices, sunscreen, alcohol use, and immunizations.[273] Physicians smoke less and make healthier food choices,[274] which isn't surprising, and almost 25 percent of doctors don't drink alcohol, and nearly half have less than one drink a week. Physicians who exercise and don't smoke are also more likely to reach blood pressure targets.[275] Want to be healthier? Become a patient of a physician who cares about personal wellness.

What about physicians' happiness? Purpose has a strong relationship to physicians' happiness. It's not about the number of hours worked, but the ability to manage the workload and a feeling of personal accomplishment, joy in work and meaningful patient relationships that matter for physicians' happiness, according to a study of 2,000 family physicians.[276]

EMOTIONS

Always trying to be perfect, never making a mistake? How about having emotions, which cloud judgment and influence decisions? "Cognition and emotions are inseparable. The two mix in every encounter with every patient," wrote Dr. Jerome Groopman in his insightful book, *How Doctors Think*.[277] In spite of common portraits of doctors as emotionless, strong-hearted superheroes, emotions dominate in medical decisions, sometimes without doctors' conscious awareness. Positive emotions are associated with a more global view of the situation and more flexibility of the decision process. Negative emotions diminish the bigger picture for the benefits of smaller details, prompting to anchoring biases (relying too heavily on one piece of information) so common in diagnostic errors.

Physicians are healers and abide by the "first do no harm" mantra, while doing the emotionally challenging work of practicing medicine, which takes a toll. Witnessing death and everyday experiences of unexpected complications, treatment failures, and patients' pain and suffering haunts physicians, causing career dissatisfaction, drug addiction, increased alcohol use, divorce, and burnout.[278,279]

Most of us remember the first death of a patient. At 59 years old, Irina Wog was tall, voluptuous, with long brown hair pulled back, a little limp—one leg shorter than the other—a loud voice and a wide smile, reflecting an optimistic outlook on life. She was admitted for an elective gynecological procedure. She came with her husband, who was the opposite: petite and quiet. He looked at Irina with puppy-dog eyes, even after almost 30 years of marriage and six children together. Irina was referred by a local gynecologist for hysterectomy with vaginoplasty.

She didn't have cancer, or any emergent indications for surgery. Her major goal was vaginoplasty, a procedure that aims to tighten up a vagina that's become loose from childbirth and aging. Indications for uterus removal or hysterectomy weren't convincing: benign uterine tumors, called fibroids. After the exam, I shared with Irina and her husband my concern that the procedure might not really be necessary. In my mind, the risks of that surgery outweighed the benefits. But that wasn't what my patient thought.

Her desire to have better intimacy with her husband, which she thought was impaired by six vaginal deliveries, seemed much stronger than the risks of the surgery. "I am healthy," she said, missing the possibility of unexpected complications. At that time, there was no informed consent concept in Russia. A verbal consent between patient and a doctor was enough to acknowledge all risks. Irina looked at her husband with a smile and stopped me, saying, "We want it to be done. We've made the decision."

The surgery was the day prior to 1st May, the Day of Peace and one of the most celebrated Russian holiday weekends. The surgery was uneventful, and Irina gave me her habitual smile, wishing me a good holiday when I visited her before leaving the hospital in the evening. Twenty-four hours later, I got a phone call from my partner that she was dead. "She got up, started walking, became short of breath and passed out. We tried to resuscitate; it just didn't work. I'm sorry."

Despair and guilt of failure on the largest scale are the feelings doctors experience when they lose a patient. Those feelings continue to be a source of emotional distress in the long term. I saw patients dying in the hospital during my training, but this was different. I couldn't breathe. For a moment I stopped hearing the voice of my colleague. "Please say it again," I said. He repeated the message. "Are you okay?" I heard. "I'll be right there," I answered, as if it could change anything. Tears came up quietly. I couldn't hold them.

My little son woke up. "Mommy, what's wrong?"

"It's all gonna be okay, honey," I said, repeating those words, not just for him, but mostly for me. I walked to the hospital thinking about every suture I'd placed, every instrument I'd counted after the surgery, every medication I'd ordered. The guilt was overwhelming. *It's my fault; I can't practice medicine,* I thought. Irina's husband was in our conference room, talking to the doctor-on-call. The tears on his face didn't stop running. He hugged me as soon as I walked in. "I told her, don't do it! You told her too!" We cried together.

The autopsy was done the following morning. I moved the sheet covering Irina's body, opening it where her hand would be, and touched her cold fingers. I remembered her strong handshake and loud laugh, and I closed the sheet. I couldn't make myself watch the pathologist doing his routine work of opening the body, removing, and weighing the organs. I was waiting for the verdict that confirmed my surgical errors. The diagnosis was clear, as expected by the doctor-on-call. My patient had died from pulmonary embolism.

You have to realize that this was the early '80s in Siberia. At that time, we didn't have the standards of these days and pre-surgical preventive strategies to prevent the development of blood clots.[280] A blood clot had provocatively traveled from Irina's deep veins in her legs after the surgery to the lungs' vessel, blocking blood flow that led to low blood oxygen levels, which caused damage to other organs in the body, including the heart. Simple compression stockings, pills or injections of a blood thinner can prevent this complication now.

My grief, and the emotional consequence of my patient's death, was overwhelming, even though at that time I couldn't have prevented it. Doctors feel guilty about a lot of things in medicine. "I wish I could have convinced my patient not to do the surgery following my initial instinct." "I wish we knew how to prevent this complication then." "I wish it wasn't me who'd done the surgery." With every death, doctors, irrespective of seniority, inevitably question the quality of care they deliver. Uncertainty about the treatment delivered can increase the emotional toll afterwards.

Nearly 80 percent of doctors reported experiencing a distressing patient event within the last 12 months and close to 40 percent suffer from depression, anxiety, and PTSD.[281,282] Every day, one doctor dies from suicide.[283]

Emotionally disturbing trauma makes every third doctor (28 percent) consider quitting or changing profession. Physicians may internalize the tragedy that happens in another family, especially if they have their own children, making themselves more vulnerable to emotional trauma. Some experienced physicians deal with difficult situations by externalizing the problem or by becoming a little numb.

Another strategy, often the subject of medical satire, is the doctors' morbid sense of humor when dealing with the most difficult trage-dies. To newcomers, this humor is initially found distasteful but is quickly learned; no one finds death funny, but it's often used as a defense mechanism.[284]

As you might have figured out, being a good doctor is not about gender, school or years in practice. It's about competence, expertise, empathy, professionalism, and interpersonal skills that meet your expectations. Be clear what your priorities are and look for someone who you can trust and rely on. Someone who listens and values your input, whose knowledge and expertise help you to make the right decisions, whose professional skills don't let you down when you are sick and who provides guidance in your health journey.

CHECK YOUR INVENTORY:

1. Make a list of the qualities that are important to you and list them in the order of priority: basic competence, expertise in the field, years of experience, Ivy League education, US medical school graduate, gender, speaks your language, availability, accessibility, social media presence, bedside manners, etc.

2. Check the social media reviews and biographies of doctors whose practices are close to your home, and identify a few doctors based on your priorities.

PART THREE

HOSPITALS

"The sooner patients can be removed from the depressing influence of general hospital life the more rapid their convalescence."

CHARLES MAYO, FOUNDER OF MAYO CLINIC

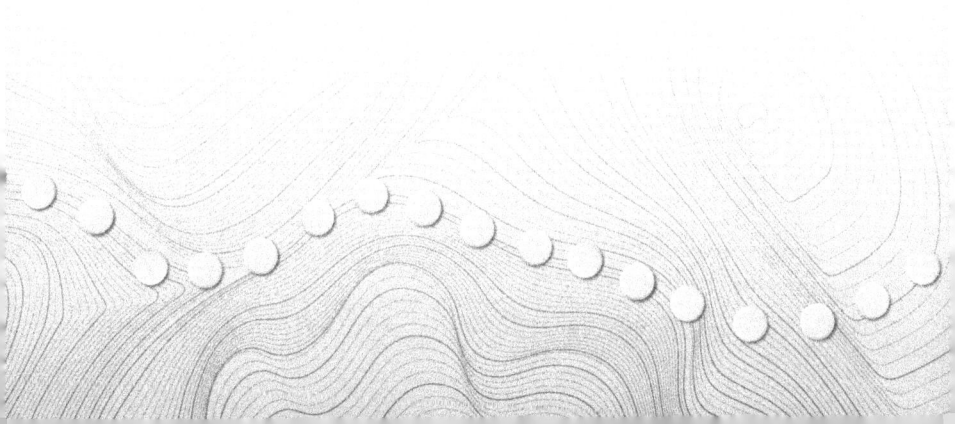

CHAPTER 20

HOSPITALS ARE "HOMES" FOR DOCTORS, BUT NOT FOR PATIENTS

The operating room's bright lamps were focused on the hole between the white sheets where blood, flesh and metal instruments were mixed in the surgeon's hand movements. More blood, less flesh, more metal instruments were inserted. Finally, there was no blood, just sutured skin. "Great work, all," I heard my mother's calm tone of voice. I couldn't see her face but recognized her figure with familiar movements in the white scrubs, a tall white hat covered by a thin white drape that also covered her face. She looked up at the amphitheater, 10 feet above the operating table, dedicated for students to observe the surgery, saw my face and made a quick movement with her eyes, signaling me to come down.

My mother was called to the hospital frequently during the evenings or at night. We had no car, but our downtown apartment was a 15-minute walk from the hospital. I remember running as fast as I could on my fast walk with my mother, with my always ready-to-go small white bag. The first "to go" bag had little dolls with clothes that eventually changed to books. "We have been called for duty," I proudly told my friends, enjoying the respect in their eyes.

The most magical room in the hospital was the operating room; a hall, as it was called because of the high dome-shaped ceiling with rows of heavy wooden benches along the walls, going up 20 feet above the operating tables. While medical students and residents watched their teachers doing surgeries from the first row, I had my own place on the top bench, which was too high to see the details of what was going on in the surgical field but let me recognize the pattern from no blood to lots of blood, more metal instruments, then flesh, then dried off and sutured skin. That was the sign that we might go home soon. I learned to recognize the nurses and doctors I met in the break room and nursing stations behind the figures dressed in all-white scrubs with tall white hats, masks and long shoe coverings that reminded me of cosmonauts.

I used to close my eyes when the flesh, separated from the body, was taken on a tray to the pathology room nearby, after the memory of a leg, amputated from the hip and taken from the human still lying on the table, had haunted me at night. Even when I'd grown up, I remembered it when I assisted an orthopedic surgeon on an amputation during my internship. My memory of the university hospital takes me home. Instead of calling a babysitter, my busy surgeon mother used to leave me in the hospital anatomy museum, next to her office, while she checked on her patients. While she hoped that I would occupy myself with children's activities involving papers and pencils, which she left in abundance on the desk, instead I made myself busy browsing the shelves of large jars full of formaldehyde-preserved tumors and disease-crippled hearts, brains, and livers, shamelessly displayed on the ground floor of the hospital.

I was fascinated by the pieces of human bodies. In the dark corner of the room there was an anencephalic fetus pressed into a large jar. It was a boy the size of a newborn. His head looked unusually cut off: he didn't have a brain. Otherwise, the boy had eyes, ears, a mouth and a content look. His eyes were peacefully closed and his lips tight. He was there every time I came in and was the only human being there to keep me company. Every time I would rush to my tiny friend to say hi, hoping that one day he would open his eyes. I used to tell him stories from my life, hoping he might smile. I felt sorry for leaving him alone in the dark when it was time for me to go home. It was the '60s, and it was Siberia. Life was different. I didn't grow up with the image of Peter Pan or Superman. There were no Barbies. The healthcare I came from was also different. But it was the same girl fascinated with the powers of medicine and almost religious gratitude to the place called the hospital—a place for miracles.

Most of us are born in hospitals. Most of us return to experience our last days there. Patients don't consider the hospital "home" though. But doctors who work there frequently do feel that way. When one is at home, there is freedom of things, actions, and time. Hospitals, for patients, are everything about the lack of autonomy. For patients' safety, medicine has become the most regulated industry. On the way to getting there, it has been separated from patients' desires, goals, and the purpose of care.

The word hospital comes from the Latin root *hospes*, meaning guest or stranger. The words hospice and hotel have the same root, connecting them to the meaning of "lodging." You might refer to the "last lodging" before permanent departure from this world, and the other as a temporary hospitality place. The other part of the root comes from *patior*, meaning "to suffer,"[285] making hospitals literally a place for sufferers to stay or a "place to suffer." Modern patients immediately imagine doctors and nurses in blue scrubs, rushing journeys with "sufferers" covered with oxygen masks or shocking them with electric currents to bring them back to life. Thankfully, the times are over where the vast majority of patients perished from infections, complications of diseases, and ramifications of treatments, and exited hospitals through the morgue. Typical thoughts about safety and discomfort while being in a vulnerable state, in hospital, have extended to concerns about the cost of that "hospitality."

HOW TO CHOOSE A HOSPITAL

When Jerry Scott, a retired nurse, was diagnosed with multiple myeloma, she knew she needed to choose a hospital for treatments and emergencies. She'd worked in a small county hospital for more than 15 years, so was familiar with the routines and hassles patients go through.

"It's a medical factory," she said to me. She wasn't alone in this definition. Lean business principles of manufacturing from the Toyota Production System—elimination of waste in pursuit of the most efficient methods—took center stage in hospitals' management some time ago.[286] David J. Yu, MD, MBA, medical director of Adult Inpatient Medicine Services at Presbyterian Hospital in Albuquerque, NM, translated this statement even further: "We see the hospital as a factory and our hospitalist group as an assembly line that is in the business of manufacturing perfect discharges."[287]

Jerry Scott didn't want to be a "widget" in the assembly line. Her expectations were simple: to be safe, to be heard, to be cared for with professionalism and compassion. With limited resources saved for retirement, she also didn't want to end up broke. This reflects most patients' expectations for healthcare delivery: quality of care for a reasonable price.[288] "I understand that healthcare is a battlefield where everything is devoted to winning the battle with illness and death," explained Jerry. She had been among "saviors" for 35 years, and now she was about to become a "sufferer." This transition didn't feel pleasant. Sufferers lie down in their beds and bear whatever illness sends them, patiently waiting for whatever saviors govern to heal with.

Three factors truly matter for the choice of the hospital besides coverage by your health plan: patient experience, safety measures and patient outcomes. Patient satisfaction is the number-one rank that I would suggest you pay attention to. Look at patient experience comments from the consumer reviews on Google, Yelp or Facebook, in addition to the hospital ranking websites. It should give you a ballpark view on the culture of safety.[289] "Word-of-mouth" is still the best marketing tool for healthcare. Patient satisfaction surveys are modern versions of word-of-mouth experiences. Check rates of re-admission, complications, and mortality (death) and length of stay in comparison with national rates. Hospitals that have a high rating in support of their staff also usually excel in patient experiences and responsiveness to concerns.

Safety measures data records how frequently patients suffer from complications during their hospital stay, such as falls, infections or surgical complications, as well as areas of expertise or additional accreditation (trauma, stroke or cancer care). Medicare, CDC, Agency for Healthcare Research and Quality (AHRQ), and Joint Commission also have a list of accredited programs. The higher the accreditation of certain care, the more trained the personnel, the better the safety procedures and the best resources. QualityCheck.org provides reliable hospital quality measures for multiple medical conditions (heart attack, heart failure, stroke, pneumonia, pregnancy, surgical care), 30 days mortality (death) rate and patient experience. On the Hospital Safety Grade website you can find scores for a hospital's overall performance from preventable harm and medical errors.

The search for a good hospital starts with determining your priorities. If you take a sick child to the hospital or deliver a baby, it's better to know that the hospital has resources, particularly intensive care beds, or beds, including ICU, for children or newborns, and therefore specialists and staff in the hospital where you are being treated. Start this process as soon as you become aware about medical conditions that may require hospitalization. It might be surgery, delivery of a baby or a chronic medical condition. If you have a life-threatening emergency, the best hospital is the closest one to you, where you can quickly be resuscitated and stabilized, which means the major vital functions of your body are restored. If you have a specialist, for example, a surgeon, who you prefer to do your surgery, you might check for their hospital privileges in different hospitals and rank those hospitals only or get the surgeon's advice. Your outpatient medical team should be able to assist you with that. Make an informed choice instead of a rushed one.

CHECK YOUR HEALTHCARE INVENTORY:

1. Look at the map for the hospitals close to your home:

    a. Which is the closest? This is the hospital that most ambulances will take you to in case of an emergency. Is this the hospital you would like to be treated in?

    b. Check social media for patients' reviews, consumer reports, your primary care doctor, consultant and your trusted circle of family and friends about this and other hospitals to choose the best option for you in case of labor and delivery, child's illness, or other medical emergency, elective surgery or treatment.

3. Share your wishes with your significant other, who will make medical decisions if you are not able to.

CHAPTER 21

HOME RULES FOR HOSPITALS

t's not a secret that people are scared of hospitals. There is merit in this fear. After the studies about the 440,000 deaths every year from preventable medical errors in US hospitals were published two decades ago,[290] preventable medical errors were considered the third leading cause of death in the US, behind only heart disease and cancer.[291] Fortunately, according to the most recent studies, by Dr. Benjamin Rodwin and his collogues from Yale University, these estimates correspond to approximately 22,165 preventable deaths annually and 7,150 deaths for patients with greater than a three-month life expectancy. The vast majority of hospital deaths are due to underlying disease.[292] Before the COVID-19 pandemic, for the first time in half a century, home surpassed the hospital as the leading place to die in the US.[293]

It seems that there are just a few things in hospital we have control of. Even if you can walk, that doesn't change the hospital rule of patients being taken in wheelchairs or stretchers for procedures and even to be discharged. Waking up for temperature and other vital-sign checks and labs at 4am and tolerating hospital noise all day and night are also hospital expectations that don't help you deal with the stress of illness. As patients, we shouldn't mind exposing ourselves, even while the door to the room is open, so our wound can be assessed, or we wait meekly for hours for the discharge papers. But there are ways for patients to make a hospital stay not only safe, but also feel "in control."

BE A TEAM MEMBER

Jerry had her own ways to be noticed. She brought silk pajamas of different colors to hospital, like she once had with her RN uniform. She wanted to express her feelings through color and communicate them clearly to all: pink for happy, blue for worried, black when in pain, purple for feeling lonely and sad. She wrote the color scheme down and put it on the bedside table and the communication board on the wall, to avoid unnecessary questions.

Despite being on the *sufferer's side*, as a patient, Jerry didn't want to be a *passive sufferer*. "I am the one who is going to pay for all the services. I want to be involved in every decision about my care." Jerry wanted to be a part of her team. There is a remarkable link between respectful treatment and patient safety.[294] Those who felt disrespected while in hospital were two and a half times as likely to experience a medical error, whether it was a hospital-acquired infection, a wrong diagnosis, an adverse drug reaction or a prescribing mistake, than those who thought they were treated well.[295] The secret is in communication. Get to know your hospital team, their roles and how to reach them. Get your special "insider ally" from the hospital team and learn how and to whom you should communicate different needs and communicate your symptoms and concerns clearly to the right team member. To be a part of your team, you should be aware of your treatment regimen or delegate this task to a family member or caregiver.

HAVE YOUR OWN ROUTINE

Jerry Scott showed her sparkling personality even at times when others succumbed to the darkness of illness. She smiled frequently, showing her missing two front teeth—a side effect of her chemotherapy. She tried to encourage and uplift the phlebotomist who struggled with her disappearing veins, her roommate who was grumpy about being woken up at 4am for blood pressure checks, or the intern who stumbled during a presentation at the team rounds.

"What is your secret to being always happy and satisfied when in the hospital?" I brought up the question that all our residents wanted to know.

"I have my own routine every day at home. I adjust it to the hospital's," said Jerry. Frequently, hospital routines, focused on safety, regulations, and efficiency, don't match patients' expectations for privacy and convenience. This is usually the experience most patients are not ready for. The good news is that things are predictable in a hospital. Being familiar with hospital routines and creating your own routine around them can give you a sense of control.

Jerry had a bright-pink notebook with gold letters on it. "My book," she called it. It was her hospital life schedule and instant companion for all doctors' visits and hospital stays. "I like my life organized in any situation with the potential of chaos," she joked. Her book held the names of all hospital staff members she had communicated with, plus their roles, location, phone extensions and even their birthdays. There were also names of pets, children and grandchildren of medical practice staff members who shared talks with her.

Every morning, Jerry made sure the hospital blinds were up to let the sun in. As a nurse, she knew that human bodies are in tune with the rhythms of the sun. With daylight, increasing levels of hormones pick us up in the early morning, then decline throughout the day, being the lowest later in the day. This is called our circadian rhythm. There is a term in medicine of "sundowning," when people, especially the elderly, develop confusion later in the day and start wandering about. The pineal gland—a tiny gland located between our two brain hemispheres—serves as a time center. It produces melatonin, which increases in the bloodstream at night, helping us sleep. Opening the blinds and letting in the sun in the early morning helps us to stay in our natural circadian rhythm, which reduces stress and gives us a better sleep during a hospital stay.

She also had tools to keep up with the hospital noise, one of the biggest stressors in hospital. A number of studies have shown that hospital noise generally exceeds the recommended level of 35 decibels (in a quiet office) and usually falls in the range of 45 decibels (room conversation) to 68 decibels (loud music heard through headphones). Noise in this range increases heartrate, blood pressure and other measures of stress. It interferes with sleep activities necessary for healing. To minimize the risk of infection, hospitals use materials such as metal, stone or tiles, which are acoustically reflective. As a result, as hospitals become cleaner, they became colder, noisier, and less comforting.[296] Jerry had her own library of audiobooks, podcasts and music streaming when she wanted to have quiet time and to spread out throughout the day at particular times when she needed distraction.

"The game is on!" Jerry announced every time our in-service team of interns, residents and medical students got to her hospital bed. We closely followed her chosen pajama color language and tried to be "on time." When she was feeling strong and was able to talk, she knew everyone by name and asked about things at home, enjoying the chat instead of talking about her failing kidney function, difficulty breathing or swollen legs. She listened to all the reports that her resident doctors presented and asked questions about the plan.

THINK POSITIVELY

One evening, when I came in to see a patient who had to be transferred to the ICU, I stopped by Jerry's room. She was lying peacefully with her eyes closed, headphones in. I didn't want to disturb her, but she opened her eyes, finishing her long breath. "Don't worry, I'm okay," she said, noticing the worry in my eyes. "I'm meditating on all the good that is still left here. I breathe positives in and negatives out." She smiled. "In and out." Jerry, like many other people with optimistic intentions, was determined to overcome her illness.

Robert Ader, American psychologist and father of psychoneuroimmunology, set up a famous experiment on classical conditioning in rats.[297] He fed them a combination of saccharin-laced water before giving them the drug Cytoxan to induce nausea and induce taste aversion. Afterwards, the rats, in spite of being fed only the saccharin-laced water, died in great numbers. Even without taking the drug, the rats' immunological system had been suppressed with the mere stress of drinking water that had previously been associated with nausea, through classical conditioning. A positive attitude will not cure, but it will definitely improve your experience with the adversities of treatments.[298] If you don't believe in positive thinking philosophy, you might choose to follow the wisdom of the alternative "not negative thinking."[299]

The truth is, you want good luck on your side when exposed to risky procedures. The "law of attraction," first described in the book *The Secret of the Ages*, by Robert Collier, has been called naïve magical thinking, bordering on delusional. But proponents of the law of attraction claim that quantum physics proves that the mind has the power to actualize thoughts via remote influences on matter. This assumption might be a misguided interpretation of quantum entanglement,[300] but is harmless enough to follow while in hospital and wishing for positive outcomes.

PAY ATTENTION

I stood up and said goodbye to Jerry. She continued to breathe in and out the happy messages to her brain. She needed her anchor to be carried away from fear. Fear is normal while in hospital because of associations of illness and death. My good friend, a former pilot, told me during turbulence on a flight, "It's just bumps in the road." These simple words provided me with a comfort of positive thinking for years ahead. I started using this expression for my patients during their hospital stays too, "It's just a bump in the road. It'll be over soon."

In our daily life, we forget about breathing, which is powerful enough to influence not only our heartbeat and blood pressure, but also our mind. We tend to breathe shallowly when anxious, asleep or in pain. Shallow breathing causes mucus to be trapped in the lungs, which increases risk for pneumonia, which is one of the most common complications of a hospital stay. Paying attention to our breath, when waking up, before a blood draw, a procedure, or before going to sleep, besides directly benefiting the lungs, will also reduce stress.

I was looking at Jerry's chest going up and down under the blanket and reflexively started breathing slower and deeper as I walked through the empty corridors of the hospital. It might have been my imagination, but I felt relieved from my worries about Jerry, my other ICU patient, myself, and my children waiting for me at home. Jerry was breathing positive messages to my world: in and out.

DOCUMENT YOUR JOURNEY

When Jerry started losing her battle with multiple myeloma, we started seeing Mary, her best friend, sitting next to her bed with Jerry's pink book in her hand. Best friends since high school, they went to different colleges, lived in different towns, got married, raised children, then lost their husbands, but never stopped being best friends. Mary moved to Summerville, where Jerry lived the year she got sick. Mary tirelessly wrote in the diary what was happening to her friend when Jerry couldn't.

Some doctors feel intimidated by patients documenting words

and actions. Transitions from one service or team to another, from the hospital to outpatient, are bottlenecks where most errors are anticipated. Doctors have their own checklists, borrowed from airline industry safety protocols, which assure that information about patients is transferred during transitions. Jerry had assigned the role of "bookkeeper" to Mary. Treatments, procedures, consults, follow-ups—all recommendations were meticulously recorded.

I made my own mistake of not following Jerry's rules of recording doctors' instructions when I picked up my generally healthy husband after an uneventful hip replacement. I didn't pay attention to the instructions the nurse patiently tried to communicate to us as I was focused on getting things together. *I'll read that later*, was in my mind. Despite decades of caring for patients after surgeries, the following morning I had more questions than answers. From the team of nursing staff to physical therapists and even food delivery, it was just me left to deal with my husband's pain, to watch for falls because of the sedating effects of pain medications. The simple task of putting pressure stockings on threw me off my feet: they had to be tight! Google and YouTube became the advisers for us, two doctors, in the post-op period.

SET YOURSELF UP FOR DISCHARGE

Hospital safety is not just about the time you spend in the building walls, surrounded by the medical staff, who're ready to step in. It's also about setting up the stage for your next steps. Some people rush home, even knowing that there isn't much help available, over-estimating their own strength.

Margaret, my 78-year-old patient, refused to go to the rehabilitation center to instead get back home to be with her husband, who had a severe form of Parkinson's disease. We set up physical therapy and an occupational therapist to come to her home after her surgery for a hip fracture and made arrangements for a hospital bed. Her children took turns to be with her. She was back with the other hip fractured the following week, after a fall while helping her husband get up at night, when nobody was there. Spending a few days in the rehabilitation unit would have been a better step for her.

Always ask for the physical and occupational therapist to visit your home right after discharge. You would be surprised by the number of good suggestions they can offer, from having the food tray at a certain place, to the toilet being raised, and answers to questions such as, when can I safely go for a walk? What medications will I be taking and when? Should I take my old medications? Is there certain food I should stay away from?

It's a common disappointment for patients when their physicians don't know about their hospital stay. "How come you didn't know?" sounds like, "Why weren't you with me when I struggled?" In spite of the efforts of hospital transitions teams, this happens more frequently than we want. Discharge summaries get faxed late or never, sometimes they aren't detailed enough or are erroneous. Hospital EMRs don't always talk to the EMR systems of doctors' practices. The solution for this problem? Be proactive. Inform your doctor about your admission. Let your doctor know about the planned discharge date and obtain all necessary documentation. Set up a visit with your primary care doctor to assure your transitions happen correctly, and you are taking the right medication and your recovery is on track.

After Jerry passed away, her friend Mary brought me Jerry's pink book. The last pages were filled with the survival tips she'd created while being admitted for complications of her multiple myeloma, which she fought with her usual fierceness. Here they are:

- Organize your life around hospital routines: let the sun in every morning; set up time for meditation and things that lift your spirit, such as podcasts, audiobooks, music lists, movies.

- Get to know your hospital team, their roles and how to reach them. Get your special "insider ally" and learn how and to whom you should communicate different needs.

- Be assertive and communicate your symptoms and concerns clearly to the right team member.

- Be aware of your treatment regimen or delegate this task to your ambassador, family member or caregiver.

- Keep an eye on your devices and tubes by asking the purpose and length of time you should have each one.

- Set a good intention. Think about your goal of being there. Establish your mantra with a few words, such as, "I'm gonna be fine," and get back to those words and the image every time fear and worry arise.

- Practice gratitude. Be grateful to your body for its resilience, your loved ones who worry and support you in this journey and extend it to the hospital staff who make you comfortable, the doctors who bring relief to your suffering.

- Focus on something other than illness, such as your breathing, meditation, book of anecdotes, or comedy, write your story.

- Treat your body as your best friend with love and kindness. "Dear friend, thank you for serving me for years. I am here."

CHECK YOUR HEALTHCARE INVENTORY:

1. Imagine that you are going to be admitted to hospital and spend a few days recovering from surgery or going through treatment. What activities and things would make you feel better that are in your control? Make a list.

2. Find your "ambassador" and discuss how you would like to be treated in hospital.

CHAPTER 22

HOW TO GET THREE DOCTORS FOR THE PRICE OF ONE

s it safe to be treated in a teaching medical practice or teaching hospital? I hear this question a lot; people want confidence, experience, and developed skills in their doctors. "Young doctors can make errors, and those errors involve real people. They struggle with lack of sleep, and they order more tests, learning to be comprehensive. *This isn't safe!* That's how you might think, but it's quite the opposite.

Approximately every fourth hospital in the US has an educational mission and is affiliated with a medical school. In a study of 21 million hospitalizations, mortality rates were found to be significantly lower in the teaching hospitals compared to non-teaching hospitals. Academic medical centers tend to accumulate attending physicians with greater expertise and greater experience. Teaching hospitals are early adopters of new and more expensive technologies, which require specialized knowledge to achieve teaching intensity and quality.[301]

Newly graduated doctors are granted temporary medical licenses for the time of their residency training, where they practice under the supervision of licensed and Board-certified attending physicians.

Every year, on 1st of July, graduates of medical schools, in new white jackets—symbols of their achievement—with name tags, and stethoscopes around their necks, as residents walk into the hospitals and medical offices for their first rotations with pockets packed with notes, handbooks and pens of different colors. They are excited, anxious, and ready for action. The first training year is called an internship and is one of the most stressful years in the life of any physician. During the first two weeks, interns go through intense orientation to the hospital, ambulatory practices, take resuscitation training courses, learn how to use electronic medical records, and prescribe medications. Two weeks later, when the thrill and confidence nurtured in medical school has drained away, and they realize the amount of knowledge and skills they don't yet have but need, the pressure of responsibility for human lives feels heavy and sometimes overwhelming.

By the end of each month, after passing a steep learning curve, the interns learn their way around the hospital, cafeteria, and the sleep rooms. Familiarity stretches into routine; the feeling of certain confidence returns. Acquired medical knowledge slowly fits into the pattern of recognition of patients' symptoms and signs of illnesses.

For over 30 years, I have been privileged to work closely with resident-physicians. The residents spend more time with a patient than the supervising physicians. They are more interested in their personal lives, families, and hobbies, which creates a special bond. Being a patient in the residency-based clinic or hospital means patients get three doctors "for the price of one." In hospital, every patient admitted to the teaching service is treated by an intern or resident, upper-level resident and attending. In the clinic, there is usually a resident and attending. Patients usually get more time with two doctors to answer their questions, to be examined thoroughly and discuss their treatment in detail.

As an attending physician in the hospital, I examine every patient individually, sometimes with or without residents, in addition to the walking rounds with the team. Twice a day, the details of admission and patients' daily progress are discussed by the whole team during rounds, where diagnoses are questioned, results verified, and recommendations are made. Every patient is examined at least two or three times, symptoms are confirmed, laboratory results are ascertained, diagnoses analyzed, and options for treatment are identified.

Resident-physicians have an ambition for a cure, they are enthusiastic and proud to finally be able to "help people." This ambition drives them tirelessly to search for answers to many of their questions and seek solutions to give hope to their patients.

Residency teaches them not only fluency to apply the knowledge they received in medical school to real patients, but also to accept that a cure is frequently not possible, though healing might be their main purpose. During residency, new doctors learn to practice their interviewing and examining skills, as well as develop analytical skills of making a diagnosis and choosing treatments. Beside mastering proficiency in procedures and surgeries, doctors learn how to connect with each individual, so people open up and tell the stories of their bodies and the way illness has changed them. They are instructed and advised by faculty on how to translate those stories into the language of anatomy and physiology, and then to come up with a diagnosis. Even when a diagnosis is reached in their minds, and only when they convince the patient to be their partner, can they accomplish the ultimate outcome. In my experience, patients appreciate resident-physicians' enthusiasm and dedication.

Dr. Lutz was anxious to start seeing patients in the clinic, as do many interns. He was tall and loud with a down-to-earth personality. He met a patient, John Walsh, in the ED during his first hospital rotation. John had heart failure and was admitted with difficulty breathing and swelling of his legs. After John was discharged from the hospital, Dr. Lutz followed up with John in the clinic. Residents discuss every patient with an attending, who most of the time goes into the patient's room to confirm history and perform physical examinations. When I walked in, and was properly introduced as an attending, I suggested making a change in John's medications. John's face became unhappy. "I don't care what you think. I'll do what *my doctor* tells me to do," he muttered and glimpsed at an embarrassed Dr. Lutz. The trust in his young doctor clearly outweighed the knowledge value of the experienced supervising physician. I couldn't have been prouder of Dr. Lutz.

Doctor Mary E. Charlson and her colleagues from Cornell University compared care provided by faculty and resident-physicians. The pattern of care for chronic diseases, such as diabetes, asthma/chronic obstructive pulmonary disease (COPD), congestive heart failure, ischemic heart disease, and depression, didn't differ between residents and attendings' patients, except that residents' patients with asthma/COPD, ischemic heart disease, and diabetes were admitted more frequently than attendings' patients. The outpatient care of residents was, on average, 30 percent more expensive than attendings, mostly driven by a higher rate of consultations and radiological procedures. Hospital admission rates and inpatient costs were slightly higher for resident-physicians. It's not surprising. Doctors who are more confident in their physical exam findings, order fewer tests, seek less consultant advice, providing more affordable care.[302] However, compared with faculty outcomes, residents' care, with dedicated supervision and additional time, result mostly in similar quality patient outcomes.[303]

There is one extra benefit of being a patient of a resident-physician. Every resident-physician must keep up with the most current knowledge to prepare to pass the specialty board exams, which require them to stay informed with the latest health information, practices, and treatments. Just ask, and they will happily share. Generally, you are in good hands with residents as doctors.

Being a patient at a residency-based practice or teaching hospital gives patients a unique opportunity to be treated by two or three physicians, spend more time with their doctor, and be a teacher of a future generation of doctors.

CHECK YOUR HEALTHCARE INVENTORY:

1. Check if you are a patient in a residency teaching practice? If your doctor is a resident, you can always ask about the year of training.

2. If you have a concern, you have an option to talk to the Attending physician in any teaching practice or hospital.

PART FOUR

MEDICAL PRACTICES

"Healing is a matter of time, but it is
sometimes also a matter of opportunity."

HIPPOCRATES

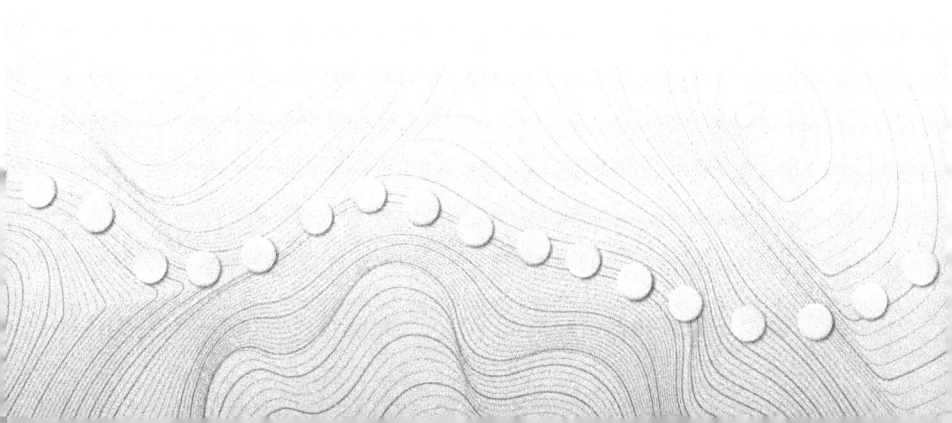

CHAPTER 23

HOW TO FIND
HEALTHCARE THAT FITS

M ommy, I'm taking Grandpa to the ER!" My daughter's voice was trembling on the phone, but something was telling me that I couldn't change her trajectory. I'd missed two messages from her while seeing patients in the clinic. "Grandpa has chest pain. Mommy, what should we do?" I heard the sound of the driving car through the phone. My 15-year-old daughter had finished her driving lessons a few weeks ago and just received her permit. *Don't panic!* I told myself, remembering how overwhelmingly anxious I was teaching her to drive.

My 80-year-old father had myriad chronic medical problems but managed to be in good health during his stay while visiting us from Russia. "Can you call the doctor to visit me?" he'd asked his grand-daughter. "I have chest pain." As a physician's kid, my daughter knew that chest pain was one of the reasons why her mother got called and rushed to the hospital. Later, she told me that Grandpa was holding his hand next to his chest, looking scared. An image she had never seen, but it was enough for her to start the mission to save him. For my dad, it was his first experience with American healthcare, and he had big hopes for it.

Primary care doctors in Russia spend half the day in the office and the other half visiting patients in their homes; those who can't come to the office, with severe pain, high fever, the elderly, homebound or families with three or four kids. Doctors make those trips by foot, with their bag packed with medical equipment and paper sheets, which, upon their return, will be inserted into the thick paper charts. Relationships with patients, their gratitude and appreciation serve as best rewards, for not only knowledge of the medicine they bring to their patients, but also the physical endurance they must have to go from floor to floor of different buildings that sometimes don't have elevators.

When I walked into the ED, I saw my dad connected to monitors, displaying his slightly elevated blood pressure, but a normal heart-rate and oxygen level. He was proudly overwhelmed by the attention of nurses, phlebotomists, and doctors. He was impressed by the efficiency, teamwork, and technology of American medicine. The x-ray machine was rolled into the small space close to his gurney and took a picture of his lungs, while an electrocardiogram was also done and monitors constantly showed the tracing of his heart.

My dad was as excited as a kid watching a spaceship about to take him into orbit. He fell in love with American medicine right there. Since that day, he became the biggest advocate for American medicine and talked about its accessibility, efficiency, and quality to all his friends back home till the end of his life. Five hours after admission, the ED doctor came in to inform us that nothing serious was going on with my dad's heart. It was confirmed that he had hypertension, an enlarged heart and he had to continue taking his medications and see his primary care doctor.

My dad thanked the doctor with tears in his eyes for saving his life, without understanding that the diagnosis was a panic attack. He just understood the word "attack," which he was saved from. A 10,000-mile trip from one continent to another was a stressful endeavor for an 80-year-old man who didn't speak English. Two weeks later, I received the bill for $17,000, blaming myself for not responding to my daughter's text messages, but reassured that my father was safe and happy.

HOW DO PEOPLE MAKE
DECISIONS ABOUT HEALTHCARE?

Apparently, this isn't always a random choice. In the late 1990s, Ronald Anderson and John F. Newman came up with a framework that explained the layman's thinking process while making choices about healthcare.[304] This decision is a function of three factors:

1. The first are predisposing factors or characteristics of who we are (age, sex, education, attitudes, perceptions), whether an individual's culture accepts the sick role or encourages stoicism, and what types of care are preferred for specific symptoms.

2. Next are enabling factors or the environment in which we live, or what is available. What hospitals, practices can we reach or afford?

3. The third is the need or why we are looking for healthcare (symptoms, chronic health conditions and how important we perceive those healthcare needs to be).

According to researchers from the Harvard T.H. Chan School of Public Health, we have a much more positive outlook on the healthcare we personally receive as patients than we do about our state or the nation's healthcare system.[305] This also means most of us in the US have been able to find suitable choices for hospitals, medical practices, and doctors. But that doesn't mean finding the right fit might not be challenging.

EMERGENCY DEPARTMENTS

About 30 percent of ED visits are potentially unnecessary, leading to an additional annual $8.3 billion healthcare spending.[306] There are reasons why ED services are that expensive. Everyone who walks in must receive a workup detailed and extensive enough to determine whether an emergency medical condition exists. What are the alternatives? Urgent care, primary care offices, online telemedicine services, pharmacy clinics, and concierge practices can provide similar primary care, with a few differences.

So, why do we choose the option of expensive, often unnecessary, services in the ER and agree to wait four or five hours in line? Primary care can be acute (outpatient and inpatient), chronic, and preventative. When we need medical care urgently or acutely, we think about an emergency room, despite the other available choices. Primary care acute office visits are different from ED visits. The latter involve more tests, monitoring, and more resources. The *Emergency Medical Treatment and Labor Act* (EMTALA) is a federal law that requires anyone coming to an emergency department to be stabilized and treated, regardless of their insurance status or ability to pay.

Comparison studies of patient and physician perceptions of the need for emergency care are close, with patients rating the urgency of their condition close to 20 percent lower than the physicians'.[307] When patients have strong connections with primary care doctors, and have an availability to be seen, they use this option first and therefore prevent about 13 percent of ED visits because of limited accessibility.[308] It's not just the perception of urgency that drives us to the expensive ED with their long waiting times though. Frequently, unsatisfied with explanations of what is being done about our health concerns, we seek "further investigations."[309]

UCLA researchers surveyed 1,100 emergency department patients. None of them had symptoms that had resulted in immediate care, and none were in severe pain or distress. More than half had spoken with a medical provider or office within the past three days and said they'd have been willing to see a doctor in a clinic instead. However, a full 70 percent reported a medical provider told them to go to the emergency room.[310] There have been many times I've told patients to go to the ER too, such as because I couldn't make timely accommodations to ensure their safety for an urgent diagnostic test or find help from the specialists, or when a patient didn't have health insurance to access certain services.

Do you have a life-threatening emergency (seizure, severe injury, difficulty breathing, very high blood glucose, or passing out)? Do you have chronic illnesses that are prone to serious complications (diabetes, heart disease, cancer, renal disease or cirrhosis), which may require hospital admission or immediate surgery? If you or your clinician believe you do, the hospital ED is the safest place to access resources necessary for life support, urgent diagnostic testing, and specialist care.

If your condition is not life-threatening, however, you would be in much better hands visiting an outpatient primary care office or urgent care. Why? EDs are not designed to provide primary care because of unnecessary testing, lack of continuity of care and high costs. Urgent care is a nice supplement for primary care, but it's not an alternative. Let me tell you why.

URGENT CARE

Kevin Gorkin came to our office with his pregnant wife, who needed prenatal care. At 34 years old, he had never had a primary care doctor after his pediatrician. "I don't need one. I eat right, I go to the gym. If I need anything, I'll walk into the urgent care next to the grocery store and get all I need, almost like a drive-through. One time, I cut my arm pretty deep and the doctor at urgent care put sutures on. They placed the splint on my leg after my ski accident. They removed a piece of wood from my eye last year. Those doctors are trained to do all kinds of small procedures, so I don't have to see specialists or go to the ER. Who wants these days to call for an appointment, then sit in the waiting room for 30 minutes to see a doctor for 10 minutes? It's not worth it for me."

Patients love the consistency of urgent care practices, having open doors for extended hours and weekends and the ability to see the same doctors and nursing staff. Many urgent-care facilities have added tele-health to the broad range of services, which has made them an excellent option for those who are otherwise healthy.

Rebecca Aronson had seen doctors at the urgent care next to her office for a decade. The warm smile from the receptionist, who always asked about her children, and the greetings of the doctors, familiar with her history without asking too many questions, gave her confidence in her care. "You've been sick a lot this year," the doctor said.

"A lot of stress, probably." Rebecca had been coming back every few months with another episode of bronchitis. Short courses of antibiotics usually made her feel better, but the cough continued. She had smoked for more than 20 years before stopping five years ago, giving herself a gift for her 50th birthday. During her last visit for "bronchitis," the doctor ordered an x-ray, suspecting pneumonia—inflammation in the lungs—and prescribed another course of antibiotics and an inhaler. She was told to come back if she didn't get better.

Rebecca was busy that summer with her garden and the grandchildren, who were out of school. The weight loss was gradual, but within three months she'd lost about 10lb, which she also contributed to being more active. When Rebecca came to urgent care with her "usual cough" symptoms two months later, the x-ray showed a large lung nodule with enlarged lymph nodes in her chest. She was diagnosed with Stage 3 lung cancer.

"It's my fault," she told me, when she came in to establish primary care on the advice of her oncologist, asking for cancer screenings and immunizations. "Doctor told me to come in if I got worse. But I didn't. I felt tired, but I attributed it to my age and stress. I saw my gynecologist for a Pap smear and mammogram. She sent me to do a colonoscopy when I turned 50. Nobody told me there was a screening test for lung cancer. I thought an x-ray I had done in urgent care was enough."

The best way the urgent care model works is by supplementing traditional primary care with guaranteed efficient acute care with less waiting time during evening hours and weekends. It is particularly suited to colds, strep throat, elevated blood pressure, acute diarrhea, urinary tract infections, burns, bug stings, animal bites, asthma exacerbation and allergic reactions, small lacerations, sprains and simple fractures.

Even if the doctors and staff in urgent care practices are fully capable of providing typical primary care and treat acute and chronic medical conditions, the workflow processes that are standardized for acute medical issues aren't intended for prevention and chronic medical problems.

CHECK YOUR HEALTHCARE INVENTORY:

1. What medical practice values are the most important for you? Rank them in order of priority.

2. Discuss with your doctor the potential scenarios when emergency department services or urgent care are the best options.

CHAPTER 24

NOT ALL PRACTICES ARE CREATED EQUALLY

With advances in medical science, and growing regulations from insurance companies, healthcare has become complex business. An African proverb says, "It takes a village to raise a child," and in the same way, even the best doctor can't do everything for you alone anymore.

My friend Susan had been following her primary care doctor for the last ten years through different practices. "I trust her; she understands me." One day, she wasn't able to reach her doctor for weeks. It made her upset. Her messages were answered, not by her doctor, but by the medical assistants. She was offered an appointment with a nurse practitioner because her doctor was booked for two weeks in advance. "I felt abandoned." Frustrated with her inability to see someone she trusted eventually made her switch to a smaller primary care practice where access to her doctor was easy.

Healthcare has become interprofessional and interdependent teamwork. When looking for a medical practice, you're not just looking for a doctor, but for an efficient and well-organized team, which will help to coordinate care between other physicians, and other healthcare professionals, physical therapists, chiropractors, respiratory therapists, psychologists, insurance companies, pharmacies and hospitals involved in your medical care.

When you seek a "doctor" these days, you will be offered to see a "provider." There are more than a million licensed physicians in the US,[311] in addition to nurse practitioners and physician assistants, who also provide healthcare services. Nurse practitioner (NP) and physician assistant (PA) roles were created in the 1960s to address a shortage of physicians and increased demand for primary care—especially in rural and inner-city settings.[312] What is the difference between providers? It takes 10–14 years of education and training to become a licensed physician, and five to six years to become an NP or PA. Primary care physicians follow the same highly structured education, guided by the Accreditation Counsel for Graduate Medical Education (ACGME), and pass the same licensure examination, with most physicians completing at least three years of supervised residency training to practice independently with broader and deeper expertise in complex cases.

Physicians spend close to 6,000 clinical hours during medical school and at least 9,000–10,000 clinical hours during three years of residency. There is no such similar standard to achieve NP certification as their educational requirements vary from program to program and from state to state. NPs start independently seeing patients after completing 500–1,500 clinical hours during 1.5–3 years of a Masters or Doctor of Nursing Practice program.[313] In specialist offices, NPs or PAs work closely with physicians and share responsibility for the patient. In primary care, NPs may have their own patient panel. Conversely, PAs must practice as members of physician-led teams and are required to be supervised by physicians in all states, although the terms and conditions vary.

What NPs have most of the time, in my opinion, is a kind and nurturing attitude toward patients, as well as more time for a visit. Patients love this and develop a strong bond with their providers, following their advice with gratitude. Multiple studies comparing the quality of primary care delivered by PCPs and by NPs and PAs generally demonstrated close outcomes measured.[314] It's always your choice if you prefer to be seen by a physician or advanced practitioner. You are the one to determine what matters: service received, timing, expertise or experience.

HOW TO FIND A MEDICAL PRACTICE
THAT MATCHES YOUR PRIORITIES

When we look for a medical practice, there are three major factors that matter:

1. Reliability
2. Convenience
3. Cost

Reliability

Reliability is about being there for you when you need healthcare. When we're ill, we're vulnerable, not just physically, but emotionally, spiritually, and often, financially too. Would you follow someone's advice and actually take the medication or take the risk of a procedure without trust? You look for a clinician who has knowledge to diagnose and treat your illness, has the skills to do procedures and find help from other services and professionals. In current, complex healthcare, trust extends beyond the doctor to the team that surrounds them. Medical practices possess your most private information, and you count on their goodwill, competence, and advocacy.

Trust itself has a therapeutic value, enhancing the efficacy of a prescribed treatment. Trust cannot be established during a rushed 15-minute visit. It takes time to develop a trustworthy partnership between patient and doctor, enough for patients to believe in the treatment plan or even understand how to follow it. Although, when doctors "run" from one patient's room to another, following a chaotic schedule of

15-minute visits, it becomes a hamster wheel that eventually leads to burnout for the clinician, potential errors, and patient dissatisfaction.

Convenience

Convenience is about being available and accessible. We don't want to drive far away, especially while sick. We look for convenient working hours and availability of different services (laboratory, x-ray, specialists) at one place. If you're a working professional or homebound because of illness, you might be interested in a practice that provides telemedicine services and efficient online communication. In efficient and well-managed primary care practices, all clinical and non-clinical staff members have assigned roles based on their expertise, training and relationship with patients to provide patients with timely healthcare services and a good experience of being welcomed, respected, your problem solved in a timely manner and to your satisfaction.

Cost

The third factor—cost—might actually be of number-one importance to you. Cost is determined by what services are covered by your health insurance and how much you're willing to pay from your pocket. For the practice leadership, cost impacts decisions about what clinicians are hired, how many patients they have to see, how much time patients spend with their doctors, and how many of the team members will work on the implementation of physicians' recommendations. Costs or profits of a medical practice will eventually determine reliability and convenience for patients.

When you're looking for a medical practice that matches your priorities, do the same as you would when looking for a partner—look for practices with similar values. Put the three deciding factors of reliability, convenience and cost in order of importance to you, and you will find what practice you are looking for.

For example, are you a healthy, busy professional, who rarely sees the doctor? Most likely then the convenience of easy scheduling, online communication or extended working hours will come first and cost will come second. If you are pregnant, the cost of prenatal care and delivery, which is usually bundled into one package, might come as a first priority with reliability second. Are you someone who struggles with chronic illness or has had bad experiences with healthcare? I bet reliability would be your number-one priority. Even for those with limited income, a reliable practice will save you money by understanding your financial limitations and by seeking the most affordable medications and services for you.

It won't surprise anyone when I say that the way a medical practice works is determined by the leadership: what services they provide, where, how, and when. This is translated into a practice's location, working hours, medical records, communication, staffing and, most importantly, the schedule. These factors ascertain patients' priorities: reliability and convenience. Remember, we're looking for a partner with similar values. A medical practice is a business, and all those factors have a common denominator: cost. Reliability of medical care with higher-salaried, more-experienced doctors, in addition to competent clinical staff, is expensive. But there is a way to cut down expenses with the implementation of modern technologies, using services of advanced medical practitioners instead of physicians, well-designed EMRs, scheduling platforms, and minimal staff training. The best medical practices have leaders who succeed in keeping a balance of the equation between factors of reliability and convenience for less cost.

So, when you look at the thousands of medical offices spread out on the map around you, how do you decide that one practice is better than another? As people are different, so are their priorities. Once you've figured out your priorities, you need to evaluate the most recommended practices to find the right fit. Satisfaction will come from meeting your expectations and matching them with the practice's values. However, there are common trends based on the ownership of the medical practice.

Traditionally in the US there are two types of medical practices: independent private practices owned by an individual or group of physicians; and practices owned by hospitals, healthcare systems, corporations, insurance or government organizations. 2020 was the first year in which the majority of physicians in the US worked outside of private practice.[315] Many small, private primary care clinics, owned by one or a few doctors, became financially strapped and were forced to turn toward external sources of funding under the pressure of the growing administrative complexity of American healthcare. This followed the trend of acquisitions of doctor-owned practices by large healthcare systems, insurance companies and private investor groups.

INDEPENDENT PRIVATE PRACTICES

Being a patient of an independent private practice owned by physicians gives you the freedom to make a choice of the doctor, hospital, and diagnostic center without ties to diagnostic centers and consultants that belong to the healthcare system. It opens doors to a bigger network of specialists, with more availability in their schedule, and potentially more feasible prices for laboratory or imaging services. Small practices implement changes quickly, they have flexibility in scheduling, working hours, workflow, and focus. Do small primary care practices provide good patient care? In spite of far fewer resources in general, small private practices are known for lower preventable hospital admission and readmission rates when compared to larger, hospital-owned practices.[316]

DIRECT PRIMARY CARE PRACTICES

Among traditional independent private medical practices, there are lesser-known membership-based, physician-owned direct primary care (DPC) practices. Patients frequently confuse them with concierge practices, immediately thinking about a high cost from the pocket. Yet DPC practices distinguish themselves from other retainer-based care models (such as concierge medicine) by charging a membership fee in place of standard fee-for-service fees, rather than on top of such fees.

DPC practices offer the full range of comprehensive primary care services in exchange for a flat, recurring membership fee, which is typically billed to patients monthly.[317] For a fee less than a telephone bill ($40–$100 based on age) for the whole family ($120) you get access to a doctor 24/7 via phone and text, and can be seen in the office when you need to be.

When I opened my DPC practice in 2015 in Summerville, SC, it was just myself and my medical assistant, who shared with me the roles of receptionist, laboratory technician, and billing service. The office looked like a vintage old doctor's home office, with bright-colored walls, decorated with paintings and books donated by my patients, and toys for kids instead of expensive electronic screens.

You might ask, how can such offices afford the luxury of longer appointments, laboratory tests, and an almost home-like environment? The answer is that DPC practices bypass the middleman; they don't bill insurance and cut down administrative expenses because they have low staffing costs. There is no need for lengthy billing-focused progress notes or staff to meet billing requirements. All time is dedicated to patients. The doctor's patient panel is reduced to 600 patients, instead of 2,000–3,000. Doctors don't spend all day in the office, but also attend patients in their office or at home when there is a need for an exam or test. Communication is direct on the phone or through texts with the goal of solving problems before coming to the office.

DPC practices encourage patients to get highly deductible insurance policies for hospital admissions and services that are not covered (pregnancy, labor and delivery, mental health). What about laboratory and imaging testing? For patients' convenience, DPC doctors sign agreements with laboratory, imaging and sometimes pharmacy facilities for cheaper cash prices.

Paired with a wraparound insurance that covers everything outside of primary and preventive care (such as emergencies and catastrophic events), membership based DPC practices might be an affordable alternative healthcare solution for families who cannot afford expensive health insurance. In some states, legislation allows the use of flexible spending accounts to pay membership fees, making this option even more affordable. However, it might not be the best choice for someone who has chronic illnesses and utilizes hospitals, rehabilitation facilities and requires frequent diagnostic testing, or someone who rarely needs healthcare.

What is in it for the doctors? Usually, it's the sense of autonomy and fulfillment from providing great quality patient care at a significantly lower cost.

CORPORATION-OWNED PRACTICES

Most medical practices that are owned by healthcare systems, government institutions or private investors are led not by physicians but by administrators, whose number is doubled in comparison with physicians and nurses.[318] Between 1975 and 2010, the number of healthcare administrators increased 3,200 percent, while the number of physicians in the US only grew 150 percent.[319]

Many new players, including venture capital investors, have entered the primary care market within the last decade, bringing focus on a consumer-friendly patient experience, modern technology, and a team approach. For example, Village MD, Oak Street, Privia Health, Crossover Health, Forward, Firefly Health, Galileo, and One Medical, recently acquired by Amazon, are primary care clinics spread throughout different states and are backed by private equity and venture capital.

Venture capital owners have introduced standardization focused on health outcomes and lowering cost, based on a data-driven multidisciplinary team approach. Their decisions are data driven, based on predictive models, algorithms, and meaningful insights on patient populations. They are the ones successfully transitioned from an old-fashioned fee-for-service model to pay-for-performance (P4P) or value-based care. In comparison with the traditional fee-for-service model—based on the assumption that the higher the volume of patients seen, number of imaging, laboratory tests and procedures performed, the higher the revenue—value-based care is rewarded for healthcare outcomes. In other words, practices are rewarded by insurance companies, corporate organizations or professional unions for lower cost of care for a *population of patients*, based on the number of chosen health outcomes.

Outcome measures also include mortality, hospital admissions, complication rates, to clinical measures relevant for chronic diseases, and patient satisfaction. While a focus on outcomes that bring "value" seems ideal, the concerns that the patients of those practices bring to light are slightly different.

In this type of practice patients have less freedom of choice to see specialists and be managed by their primary care doctor instead, or be offered to take low-cost medications, instead of costly, but more effective drugs to reduce cost of care in exchange for many conveniences offered: longer visits, having a health coach or free transportation to the office, specialist or laboratory.

Value-based practices frequently contract certain specialists and hospitals based more on cost than necessarily on quality. Be ready for the concept of "interchangeability" hidden behind the team approach. You might be offered services of a "team member" whose skills and knowledge does not match the complexity of your illness. Treatment options also might be limited to the cost-oriented priorities. You might be offered free Uber rides to see a healthcare professional but be limited in the diagnostic procedures or opinion of the consultant who could improve your suffering.

If costs are controlled by someone else, not you, would it be reasonable to believe that you will receive services that serve the goal of saving on healthcare for "populations"? What if you decide that your value is bigger than that chosen for the population? What if your measures of the outcomes are different from those of your healthcare plan or corporation? Then this type of practice is not for you.

Medical practices owned by hospitals, healthcare systems or insurance companies usually have a modern look and are well advertised; they can afford it. They also have standardized workflows to make management easier for administration and to create more revenue. They also have measurable quality and efficiency standards established by corporate leadership. Most of them are also based on the fee-for-service reimbursement model, where they are frequently rewarded with additional payments for meeting outcomes for prevention: screenings for colon, breast and cervical cancer, screening and treatment of depression, control of diabetes and hypertension.

Seven out of ten physicians are now employed by hospitals, healthcare systems and large corporate organizations.[320] By signing contracts, they are obligated to follow their employer's regulations and workflows. Every doctor's minute counts for the revenue in the fee-for-service model. Most of the time, your phone call will be answered by the phone operator, who doesn't know you and is located in a centralized office, maybe even in another state. Your information will be passed electronically, with uncertainty about who and when they will call you back.

Hospitals and healthcare systems own the practices and determine the schedule, workflow, and scope of care. They hire providers (advanced practitioners, NPs and PAs) and physicians, and pay a more or less predictable salary, usually based on the number of patients seen and on meeting established quality metrics. The drawbacks are lack of physician autonomy, limited influence on the schedule and work-flow, as well as a limited referral network. Physicians usually have a limited influence in the clinical processes that are standardized and managed by medical administrators. Clinicians have a limited role in their scheduling, staff to work with, including their professionalism and training. Work processes are usually standardized by administrators, or with minimal leadership clinician involvement. But physicians still have full responsibility, including legally for each patient, even if they can't control patients' access to care, timeliness of testing or consultations. Responsibility for patients' care without the authority to make changes in the process of treatments and practice workflow is a common reason for clinicians burning out, leading to high turnover.

So, who might benefit from these practices? Patients with public payers, who have low copay, who have chronic medical problems and need follow-up visits and regular testing, and who utilize specialists and hospital services, and may take advantage of hospital networking benefits of shared medical records.

The cons are that you might wait longer for appointments with specialists and primary care doctors because the number of them and locations are limited to the practices owned by the healthcare system. You might need to drive further from home to do the tests or procedures to facilities owned by the system. Your messages through the patient portal might be answered by people who don't know you. Your doctor might not even know about your messages. There might be reluctance and barriers for you to see specialists outside the health system; after all, who likes to promote competitors and lose clients by sending business elsewhere?

CHECK YOUR HEALTHCARE INVENTORY:

1. When you are looking for a medical practice, recognize which are the independent private practices, hospital/healthcare network-owned practices, direct primary care practices, and concierge medical practices close to your home.

2. Match your priorities (reliability, convenience, cost) with their advertised values.

CHAPTER 25

HEALTHCARE CHOICES HINGE ON WHO WE ARE

According to studies, the attitude and satisfaction we have with primary practices seems to hinge on what generation we are from. From generation X to baby boomers, perspectives on healthcare are said to be age dependent.[321] However, it's not enough anymore for doctors to provide high-quality patient care, and, regardless of the generation, today's patients have become consumers of healthcare services, who want the convenience of scheduling appointments, timely visits, communication of choice, and accessibility outside office hours, in addition to clinician expertise.

GENERATION Z

The assumption that generation Z, or young adults born between 1997 and 2012, are generally healthy as a population has been proven wrong by studies in North America,[322] Europe[323] and Canada.[324] When transitioning to adulthood, kids experience a lot of stress and loneliness, peer pressure, and have a tendency to become engaged in risky behaviors,[325] substance abuse, and unhealthy eating habits.[326] Close to half of young adults don't have a primary care physician. This isn't because they don't need one.

Rachel Hill, 19, was dressed in clothes that sent a message to the universe that she did not hide: "I don't care" was written on her t-shirt. She changed her doctors frequently. "I don't like doctors ..." she started without keeping eye contact. "They don't answer my messages when I need help. They discharge me after I've missed appointments. Sometimes I can't get up in the morning. Just can't." Rachel had an eating disorder. She weighed 95lb and kept losing weight. She suffered from depression and had been admitted to many rehabilitation centers all over the country. She couldn't hold down a job but had written two books and had a pretty realistic view of her illness. She had a large social media presence and posted frequently on Twitter and Instagram.

Most young adults have grown up with the internet and social media as their major communication tools. They are attracted to the convenience provided by practices that offer access online,[327] telemedicine appointments, online scheduling and access to their data. They are also much less satisfied with primary care provided in usual practices in comparison to older adults.[328]

Rachel Hill didn't trust doctors. Obsessed with her thinness and a fear of gaining weight from prescribed antidepressant medications, she had a habit of stopping them. This was followed by an emotional rollercoaster and the withdrawal symptoms that exacerbated her illness. In addition to her electrolyte abnormalities, vomiting, stomach pain, dizziness, and malnutrition from the eating disorder, these symptoms were reasons for her frequent admissions to local hospitals and were followed by lengthy rehabilitations.

Generation Z don't want old-school healthcare, where they don't have input into decision-making; they want to be in charge. They will stay with doctors who communicate in their language, give them a feeling of trust, are patient and creative in explaining how the healthcare system works, let them know what their rights are and what services are available to them.[329]

It took time with Rachel to establish mutual rules and expectations. "What do you like to do?" I asked.

"Play video games," she replied.

"Do you know the rules, how to play?"

"Do I look like a dummy?"

"Our practice also has rules. If you follow them, you might like us too."

"We'll see."

We worked as a team, educating Rachel on our practice's capabilities and expectations.

"You're not there when I need you," she said early in the process.

I explained that she could send a secure message to the practice electronically 24/7 about the way she was feeling, but we would discuss the issues—unless it was a healthcare emergency—during regular, scheduled appointments, initially every week, then every two weeks. We committed to address the list of her "concerns" during those appointments.

In three months, Rachel moved to appointments every month, and the number of nighttime electronic messages decreased. She kept her promise and didn't stop medications without talking to us first, giving us a chance to convince her about their benefits. Every time she was admitted to the hospital, we followed up with her, making sure that she didn't feel abandoned and that she knew we cared.

When my 17-year-old daughter went to college, the last thing she wanted to talk about among all the new things in her life was her new doctor. Based on the experience of college girls coming to my office, I decided to give her a few choices of practices next to her dorm, instead of recommending a physician. Kids want independence and she appreciated her freedom of choice. She googled potential candidates and chose a young female doctor, whose bio had the same interests as hers and she liked her Facebook page.

After her first visit to her new doctor, she stopped asking me questions, which made me concerned initially, but she reassured me that, "my doctor explained things and gave me websites to read." Based on the insurance paperwork I received, my kid had done all the preventive testing that she needed, and I stopped worrying. The formula of effective communication, trust and continuity of care had proven to be right, and my daughter learned to look for those qualities in her doctors ever since.

GENERATION Y

Generation Y, or millennials (born between 1981 and 1996), are a healthier generation. More than half of millennials visit a doctor less than once a year. Only 35 percent engage with a primary care doctor. Money is not the issue. They value the money they spend on healthcare, and even more, they value the time assigned to it. Some 23 percent of millennials belong to the wealthy and affluent market, with at least $100,000 in investable assets.[330] Most millennials appreciate practices that are accessible, affordable, technologically advanced, and solve their problems efficiently. They realize quickly when scheduled visits are more beneficial for the doctor than them, to assure that the condition has improved or explain the laboratory values, and they don't like to waste time on follow-up visits, expecting information and advice to be delivered electronically and for technology to save them time and money.

Some 93 percent don't schedule preventive doctor visits. They are more likely to self-diagnose (28 percent) and take health-related actions, such as trying a new diet, taking a dietary supplement, changing their exercise routine or trying an alternative treatment based on information they've read on social media,[331] before going to the doctor.[332]

They look for doctors and practices with positive reviews on social media. They like to only pay for necessary services and feel comfortable to ask about prices. In comparison with baby boomers, they don't seek a close bond with their clinicians and steer toward urgent-care practices with telemedicine presence or extended hours that fit their busy lives.

Dissatisfaction with a service is a primary reason why millennials leave practices. They are an instant-gratification generation and tend to make their decisions quickly. Just one negative experience can make them switch practices by going somewhere they find more respect for their time and better "retail or customer service."[333] Medical practices compete and seek more millennials for similar reasons of time saving, efficiency and more revenue. Most millennials are healthier, they require less time for visits, have fewer hospital admissions, fewer referrals and less paperwork and clicks while filling out medical records, which is less work for doctors and less follow-up for the office staff. Millennials would rather choose primary care doctors who help with lifestyle changes, prescribe fewer medications, and are available quickly and electronically to answer their questions.

A modern, technically-savvy medical office, with available, efficient, same-day appointments, telemedicine opportunities, focused on wellness, and a practice that values their business and time would be the best choice for gen Y.

GENERATION X

Born between 1965 and 1980, generation X are called the "latch-key generation" as they were often left unsupervised at home after school until their parents came home from work. They sandwich between millennials and baby boomers and have learned the power of lost values after the global financial crisis of 2008. They grew up with the development of a strong retail culture, carry more credit card debt, and like advisers with expertise. They have reached their high peak earning, living on the cusp of midlife crises, and approaching menopause.[334]

Generation X is also the first generation that grew up in an era of available internet-based health information, direct consumer advertising, and the AIDS crisis. This generation is accustomed to being involved in the health decision-making process and health advocacy. The health behaviors of gen Xers have shown increased levels of anxiety and depression, obesity with early development of its metabolic complications, and probability of heavy drinking.[335]

Gen Xers highly value their time and expect respect for their goals and wishes. They also make decisions for their children and their parents. Being knowledgeable and capable of searching for information, gen Xers seek high-value service, expert practitioners, convenience, and ease of medical care for a reasonable price. Most of the time, they search for professionals with certifications in their fields of interest (integrative medicine, sports medicine, and evidence of excellence in the outcomes). They want more early or late appointments, after-hours, and weekend physician availability. Technically savvy, gen Xers use mobile apps to help take care of their health.[336]

Gen Xers spend time looking for a doctor with expertise and like to bring the whole family along to make communication easier. Doctors who openly talk about saving money on medications and discuss alternative treatments, involve them in decision-making by sharing the reasons for laboratory testing and imaging, and educate by pointing out available scientific evidence, usually win their hearts. They would leave a practice if they had a problem communicating directly with a physician, waited too long for appointments or noticed billing errors.

BABY BOOMERS

Baby boomers, born between 1946 and 1964, are known as a generation of self-realization, self-actualization, and self-help. They are the ones who joined protests against the Vietnam War, loved rock 'n' roll, and drove Mustangs and Corvettes with cigarettes in their hands, looking cool. Baby boomers' priorities in healthcare have developed during a time of major medical discoveries and internet availability with improved access to technology. These advances have contributed to longer life expectancy, in spite of multiple chronic medical problems. They have also managed to acquire the load of chronic illnesses. By 2030, every fourth boomer will live with diabetes, every third will be obese, and every other will find themselves suffering from arthritis, while more than half will seek out treatment options for other multiple chronic disorders.

Baby boomers have to prepare for four key "aging shocks": cost of prescription drugs, the cost of medical care that is not paid for by Medicare or private insurance, the actual cost of private insurance, which partially fills in the gaps left by Medicare, and the cost of long-term care.[337]

Overwhelmed by economic burden and mistrust of Medicare, boomers are ready now to invest in healthy aging to avoid major disability hurdles down the track. They seek advice on lifestyle modifications, supplements, new technologies, and preventive screenings, which Medicare doesn't cover. They are also more likely to debate with their doctor. Practice choice? Medical offices that are focused on their generation's priorities: good communication online, clinicians with proven expertise, who can spend time answering questions about lifestyle changes, healthy aging, and who understand financial challenges. Health coaches, such as One Medical's Practice for Seniors and small private practices, fill the gap, helping baby boomers navigate through challenges of healthcare.

SILENT GENERATION

The silent, or greatest, generation is defined as people born from 1928 to 1945. Old-fashioned, traditional medical care attracts them more than advances of telehealth and other online components of medical care. They want longer visits with their clinicians, with updates on their lives, and feel uncomfortable with online technologies. They are more likely to follow doctors' orders and defer researched information in favor of their physician's opinion. They bring gratitude and appreciation for small steps that staff and clinicians make for them by scheduling visits at convenient times and seeking transportation options. Practices focused on geriatric care, health coaching and value-based services similar to the Senior services at One Medical—formerly Iora Primary Care and recently purchased by Amazon—or private practices serve this purpose. Baby boomers and members of the silent generation are the highest users of healthcare. They are also the most challenging group, who seek high levels of medical expertise and customer service.

CHECK YOUR INVENTORY:

1. Put your priorities in order: cost, reliability, accessibility.

2. What generation do you belong to?

3. Compare your priorities with the generational healthcare values. This will help you to find a practice that is a good fit for you.

PART FIVE

ILLNESS

"Out of your vulnerabilities will come your strength."

Sigmund Freud

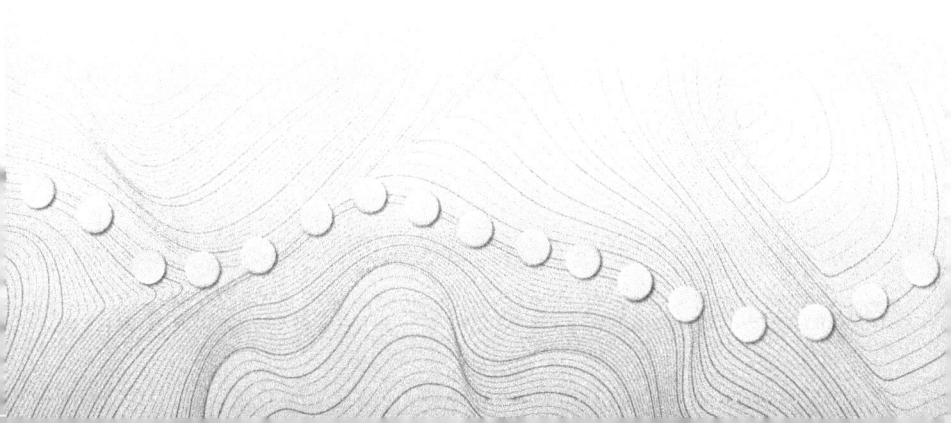

CHAPTER 26

CHRONIC ILLNESS AS A PIVOTING POINT

Physicians like to come up with diagnoses. You feel as though you've solved a puzzle with a bigger meaning: the solution of a patient's problem. Bingo! Excitement from solving the diagnostic puzzle is usually not the experience that is shared by a patient. "The good news is that we now know you have lupus. The bad news is that it sucks!" There is nothing enthusing about this for a patient. Just a road without end, sometimes even a maze. By diagnosing chronic illness, we invite patients into a lifelong journey that they didn't want and didn't plan to go through. We, as doctors, owe our patients showing the way through it, the "road map" from that pivotal point to the future.

Harry Koritz was a manager of a local supermarket. He'd worked there for more than a decade. His job was his pride and joy. At 55, Harry looked a little heavy and stocky. His dark mustache and glistening hair reminded me of Ned Flanders from *The Simpsons*. A perfect gentleman, Harry was polite, with a smile ready on his face, and always impeccably dressed in his tan slacks and red collared shirt. Harry was ready to help everyone. He used to come to our Family Medicine Center for his yearly physical to get a clean bill of health, as a stamp of his achievement—"life is good."

"Harry, your blood pressure is slightly elevated."

"This is only when I come to see you, Doc. You make me nervous. I feel great."

During the last three years, Harry had gained 12lb, the result of having a beer or two every night for stress relief. He'd also added another cup of coffee at noon to deal with his fatigue. Two weeks later, Harry came with his wife and showed the log with blood pressure measurements I had asked for, all above the normal range. Harry liked order; being "out of order" didn't fit in his life's script.

Judy, Harry's wife, wore a white dress with sunflowers on it; a look of everything in life being perfect. On that day, I diagnosed Harry with three chronic illnesses: hypertension (elevated blood pressure), hyperlipidemia (elevated cholesterol), and early onset of diabetes.

"How can I be sick if I feel well? It's probably an error. Let's repeat the labs and blood pressure measurements."

Harry's wife kept her eyes down as I could read what she wanted to say if she kept eye contact. Then she looked at Harry and started talking. "Harry, tell her…"

We both waited. It was a pause, but it didn't feel heavy. It seemed as if pressure from keeping "the secrets in the jar" had come off. "My father had diabetes and high blood pressure. He died from a stroke after spending the last two years in our house, half-paralyzed. I grew up seeing him helpless with his growing disabilities, struggling to keep up with his jobs to support our extensive family. Just the thought of being sick makes me shiver." Harry thought about his fears of being disabled and losing his job, not being able to support his family.

A DELAYING GAME

Chronic illnesses don't strike at once. There may be no symptoms for a while, or just those of, "I'm not feeling well," "I'm tired," "I can't sleep," "It's my weight," or "Too much stress." We always find excuses for those. "It's just stress at work, I need a vacation," or "I need an extra cup of coffee, that's all," or "I need a drink."

It usually takes months or years before our body fails our self-healing resources. The human body is a fascinating self-regulatory machine adapted to natural repair and recovery. As soon as tissue damage happens, your body begins the healing process to maintain its stability or balance of ideal physiological parameters: temperature, oxygen, fluid balance, acidity, and many others. When a stressor challenges the homeostatic balance in the body, mechanisms attempt to restore it.

"If the body is so good at self-healing, then why do we get sick?" asked Dr. Weil, founder and director of the Arizona Center for Integrative Medicine at the University of Arizona College of Medicine, in his book *Spontaneous Healing*. Sometimes, circumstances of imbalance and external forces exceed the capacity of the healing system, leading to failure to restore balance.[338] If those forces, such as viral load during a viral illness, tissue damage from an injury, myocardial infarction, cancer, or bacterial overload during inflammatory processes are too powerful, or occur too fast, the healing forces of the body can't be mobilized with enough speed to balance the impact. When your body persistently initiates its regulatory adaptation mechanisms for a long time, the stress response becomes more damaging than the stressor itself. That's what happens during chronic illness.

We don't want to know about chronic illness. Patients frequently come to a new doctor and intentionally don't disclose the presence of diabetes or hypertension. As changes in the body are noted as suspicious for chronic illness, what do we do? First, we deny any possibility of it by ignoring the symptoms and, instead, look for alternative explanations.

His new diagnoses surprised Harry. How did he not know about his elevated blood pressure or weight gain? The truth was: he didn't want to know. It was something he couldn't control. We deny insidious symptoms and try to cover signs of discomfort by all available means, waiting for annoying symptoms to go away. We get angry with our spouses nagging about alcohol, smoking or eating junk food.

We miss doctors' visits. We bargain, considering ourselves healthy to a level where we can get the most from our lives.

Why? Identification with illness brings fear of change, vulnerability, and death. Facing a long-lasting illness threatens our personhood and triggers recognition that our time is limited. It brings us face to face with our body's limitations and assigns a clock to our dreams and the roles in life we hoped to play. Anticipatory stress, which isn't as powerful as the stress of discovering a chronic illness, still activates the stress response out of fear or expectations of non-existing complications. It leads to anxiety and sometimes depression. Depression affects close to every fourth patient with chronic disease. The more chronic illnesses patients acquire, the more likely anxiety and depression will affect them. Besides chronic illness, depression surges affect the pro-inflammatory and metabolic factors and neuroendocrine system, leading to more pain, symptom burden and functional impairment. It affects adherence to the treatment regimen, deteriorating lifestyle habits, and, eventually, risk of death.[339]

Chronic illness brings to the surface feelings of pain, exhaustion, loneliness, disappointment, and loss. Swiss psychiatrist Elisabeth Kübler-Ross, in her book, *On Death and Dying*,[340] introduced five stages of grief: denial, anger, bargaining, depression, and acceptance. These patterns of loss have been applied to many changes in life, including chronic illness.[341] Chronic illness transforms lives entirely. As with any change, it's met with resistance and fear.

As Harry told me, "It's just you, Doc! It's just stress at work." Then we become angry and miss the doctor's appointments, argue with a nagging spouse. Some people try to find their way through the symptoms (bargaining) by trying vitamins, energy drinks and herbs that helped a neighbor, without dealing with the cause. As a result, we delay acceptance and, therefore, treatment.

Chronic illness is a process. The way you're going through it can be different to others. Even surrounded by adversities, you always have a choice either to continue taking the long road through the stages of loss of a certain part of your health, or you can accept your health as a changing path, step in and deal with the reality of your situation. "Each moment is a choice. No matter how frustrating or boring or constraining or painful or oppressive our experience, we can always choose how we respond," wrote Dr. Edith Eva Eger in her memoir about surviving Auschwitz, *The Choice: Embrace the Possible*. What is possible when we are sick with illness that will stay? This is a question we have to explore individually day by day, seeking joyful moments in life. The smell of fresh coffee in the morning, the sound of your laughing child, a beautiful sky above you or the story that you could not stop reading. Instead of ruminating on the symptoms, intentionally choose to center on feeling pleasure from the life around you.

AVOID SELF-SABOTAGE

My father, Vladimir, came from a family of eight children in rural Siberia. Five children died in infancy. There were no doctors for hundreds of miles from the village of Solonovka, in the Altai area. They had one horse that also had to be sold so they could buy food. Vladimir's parents had three years of church elementary school education. His parents didn't understand his desire for education beyond high school. There was no money, and the family needed a young boy to work on the farm instead. One day, he left the house early in the morning, way before dawn, so as not to be seen, and walked to the train station in the dark to catch the train that stopped there for only two minutes. He came to Tomsk on the roof of the train to get into law school. He not only graduated from law school but became one of the prominent political figures in Tomsk.

He blamed the harsh Siberian environment, a stressful job, long working hours, and food that was more a "surviving" source for most of his chronic medical conditions: hypertension, prediabetes, high cholesterol, heart failure, atrial fibrillation, and arthritis. Dad wasn't prepared for obligatory retirement from his political leadership job at the age of 55. "Until a certain age, we don't think about health, like it's supposed to be there for us as the sun never fails to come up every morning," he told me. "We overexpose ourselves to all kinds of risks until we get really sick. Don't continue sabotaging your health when you get hit by the burden of illness! Why? It's not death that's scary. Years of struggle while unable to live fully are worse. Don't sabotage your death!"

It might be scary to look inside of that emptiness that prompted us to start some of our habits of emotional eating or reaching for cigarettes. But it's the first step for healing—to look at your habits and identify the triggers that may be sabotaging your health.

Do you remember when and how the first cigarette became an everyday necessity? When one drink stopped being enough to feel good? Feeling pleasure is essential for wellbeing. When we don't feel pleasure or stop wanting it, it's a sign of depression, anxiety or fear. When desire comes, we want it fulfilled. We want to feel good, not in a week, month or year. Now! Desire for immediate satisfaction because of a burst of short-lived and powerful pleasure chemicals that interact with pleasure systems of the brain, bringing short-lived but intense pleasure, generates a reward–behavior cycle.

My good friend, also a physician, who fully understands the benefits of healthy eating and an active lifestyle but eats fast food pretty regularly and avoids physical activity entirely, once told me, "Growing up, the biggest reward for me was sharing a burger after the football game with my father. Everyone around me loved to play group sports. We didn't learn to exercise alone, go to gyms. We played basketball, football, and raced against each other. Now, I come home from work already exhausted. Am I going to play basketball? My wife and kids are waiting for me. I just need something quick and easy for myself."

Childhood experiences shape not only "soul foods" but also comforting behaviors focused on joy and survival because of the traits of generations before us. In the early stages of destructive habit formation, our bodies more or less handle the impact of those negative actions. As a result, our brain reward systems get confused. We receive pleasurable feelings without negative feedback from the body, which continues self-healing and sends us deeper into the motivational trap. Lack of an effective feedback system leads us to perceptual errors. Inner forces that drive human motivations to unhealthy and self-destructive behaviors are focused on basic survival instincts developed by generations of our ancestors. They bring forth actions that are followed by powerful feelings of pleasure or pain.

The human brain quickly catches the positive or negative feedback of reactions and learns to follow the pathways that generate pleasurable feelings and avoid those that cause pain in any form. Experience of immediate pleasurable sensations results from the release of endorphins and the chemical dopamine, which interacts with pleasure systems in the brain. Dopamine serves as a motivational signal for the brain to recognize pleasure, making you want more of it. This path from the action that generated the pleasure reaction becomes so powerful that it might send people onto the "hedonic treadmill."[342] People adapt to each level of pleasure quickly, looking for higher increments of pleasure, failing to sustain that feeling of happiness. Fortunately, evolution has also equipped us with less-powerful but longer-lasting feelings of joy and happiness, caused by the release of other neurochemicals (serotonin), interacting with mood-regulating centers in the brain.

Physical activity, as much as you can tolerate at that moment, has the power of bringing pleasure. We don't feel immediate satisfaction by doing 30 pushups. Quite the opposite. We get discouraged quickly from muscle pain and exertional fatigue and may stop an activity that doesn't bring intense feelings of pleasure. Psychological and physiological changes of physical activity, including mood state changes and "exercise-induced euphoria" are not that intense, but last longer, giving the feeling of satisfaction and happiness.

Does the knowledge that something is good or bad sway people enough to change their self-destructive behavior? The answer is no, according to the research studies. The desire for cigarettes and the pain of not having one becomes more powerful than the fear of risks associated with smoking.

IDENTIFYING TRIGGERS

Joan Kroger was 56. Her gray hair was always well groomed, as were her perfectly manicured nails. For the last 20 years, she'd worked as a science teacher in a local high school. Joan raised successful children, who'd graduated college, and her husband of 35 years adored her. She ate well and exercised regularly, almost as if she had to compensate for her one bad habit. She'd smoked for over 40 years. "I know, I know, it's bad for me," she used to say, smiling apologetically. "But when I get into my car, I can't stop myself. I just light up the cigarette and it feels good. I can't stop it."

I didn't expect Joan to stop smoking the same day she was diagnosed with lung cancer, but she did. Joan was lucky, even in her illness—the cancer was caught early. After the removal of part of the lung and radiation, she received the verdict that she was cancer free. Joan had wanted to cure her cancer and so stopped smoking. Her goal was to fight cancer. When she was told she was cancer free, her goal was accomplished. Three months later, she was back to her habitual cigarettes to calm herself down.

Studies of habits have revealed that success with battling bad habits has little to do with goals. Goals are results you want to achieve. Instead, habits have nearly everything to do with the systems or processes that lead to results.[343] Instead of focusing on the outcomes, trying to change as an individual will bring longer-lasting results. "I'm not a smoker." "I will be healthy." "I'm a fighter." To change your identity, you'll have to look deeper within yourself. What are your internal triggers? What surroundings, or external triggers, push you toward the immediate need of pleasure.

Joan's internal triggers were feeling anxious, sad or being alone. The external triggers were seeing cigarettes and driving. For each trigger, I asked Joan to come up with an alternative that could distract her and switch to a different feeling. We wanted to separate the habit of smoking from the trigger feeling. She left cigarettes in a more difficult-to-reach car compartment and left gum easily available. She made icy cold water available for when she was anxious and let her best friend know that she would text or call when feeling lonely.

"The biggest impact on me," said Joan after 12 months of not smoking, "were the words 'I have the power.' I kept telling myself that like a mantra every time I wanted to smoke. Feeling powerless seemed worse."

"Nothing is a faster teacher," Kübler-Ross noted, "than suffering. The more we suffer, the earlier the spiritual quadrant opens and matures."[344] Feelings of pain or loss are an even stronger driving force than pleasure. The emotional discomfort of losing $100 is stronger than the pleasure of gaining $100. Anthropologists explain this through evolved emotions, which may have foiled people's efforts and kept our ancestors on track toward long-term happiness.[345] Painful experiences may help us to stay away from habits that sabotage health and give us strength to try new, healthy ones, just to avoid them.

POSITIVE INTENTIONS

Rebecca Zimberman, a lovely librarian, had a dream. She had never been to Europe. Finally, the moment had come, and she was excited about her upcoming Mediterranean cruise—a retirement gift to herself. She spent months clothes shopping and choosing the excursions she was going to take. Before retirement, she wanted to do all preventive screenings her insurance would pay for. One of them was a mammogram, which came back showing calcifications and a small mass in her right breast. She listened quietly to the results of the breast biopsy. The breast cancer had spread to her nearby lymph nodes. She had never been married or had children. She kept herself busy with her work and being involved in the lives of her nieces and nephews. Despite her extra weight, she was relatively healthy.

She'd worked in the library for 30 years and was saving for early retirement. "When I retire, I will travel, go to the gym, eat right and maybe even date," she'd been telling me over the years. The cancer made her angry. "I'm gonna beat it. I've waited for my 'time' for so long. And I'm still gonna go on the cruise," she added, wiping away her tears. "Right after chemo, even if I have to wear a wig. I might even look better with a wig."

Rebecca underwent surgery and chemo, joined support groups, and targeted her lifestyle with precision. "I cleaned out all the boxed, processed food from my pantry. I eat mostly vegetables, fruits, and wholegrains. It's never been my favorite, but I took cooking classes and learned to cook the way I like it." She discovered water aerobics and a power yoga practice and lost almost 50lb. "I wasted so much time. I could have done all of this much earlier. I know that the medicine I take to prevent recurrence may weaken my bones, but guess what, weightlifting helps my mood and my bones." Her spirit was contagious.

It's not the illness itself, or fear of it, that motivates people to maintain efforts to conquer the challenge. Switching focus to an emotionally significant, positive intention provides the mindset that drives change. "There should be a better life than just going from one doctor to another and taking pills," my dad kept telling me.

The year my son was born, he wanted to make his first grandson a memorable gift and carved a little bunny from a piece of pinewood. That tiny bunny sparked a woodcarving passion in my father. He lived till age 82, being physically active till the last hour by carving wood, drawing sketches, creating more than 150 pieces of art that have been displayed in museums, the governor's mansion, and city libraries.

Peter Kohl was a police officer. He smoked from age 15, despised the gym and loved fast food. "My job is stressful 24/7, smoking calms me down. I walk more steps at work than any of those guys in the gym. Food is the only joy I have time for. Let it be what I like." At 42 he suffered his first heart attack. Peter stopped smoking for two years but allowed himself the occasional cigarette or two. ("I take aspirin, it'll take care of the rest.") His weight kept creeping up. He couldn't run down the stairs and settled for a desk job. "Now I'm in charge of 22 officers. It's more responsibility, more stress."

When he reached a surprising 286lb and a BMI of 38, his wife sent him to see me to check out his snoring and episodes of gasping for air at night. Severe sleep apnea was the conclusion of the sleep study. "Doc, I'm not wearing this mask to sleep, it suffocates me." Our conversations about weight loss, walking and stress reduction didn't make a difference. "I feel great. Why do I have to eat what I don't like or do something I hate? Life's too short." What he agreed to do was take his medications, the number of which grew to a list of 11 at age 56 and included three medications for blood pressure, one for cholesterol, two for diabetes, two for arthritis, one for sleep, one for depression plus aspirin. He counted on medications to do the job, more than on his own efforts. That was the only sacrifice he was willing to make.

After one long and stressful day, he developed chest pain. Cardiologists in the hospital determined there was a complete blockage of his major heart arteries. At 60, Peter had a quadruple bypass. However, life sent him an extra challenge. He suffered a stroke during the surgery. He woke up after surgery without the ability to move his right side. His body had failed to control blood flow to the brain during cooling and rewarming, necessary to prevent organ damage during cardiac bypass surgery. During rewarming, an autoregulation mechanism that protects the brain from fluctuations in the body's blood pressure malfunctioned.[346] The risk of stroke grows with patients' complexity.[347]

Recovery was long and painful. He had to retire from the job he loved and had devoted almost 40 years of his life to. His depression symptoms worsened. Peter was angry with his life, doctors and more with himself.

I didn't see Peter for 12 months, thinking he had changed doctors. He didn't return our calls. When he walked into my office, I barely recognized him, with a slight limp, 30lb lighter, smiling a broad smile. Peter looked happy and content. His blood pressure was normal, his blood glucose measure was in the range of prediabetes, and he'd reached his cholesterol goal numbers. We all wanted to know who and how Peter had fixed his health. "Miracles happen," he told us proudly.

Together with his wife, he'd had to get custody of his three-year-old grandson, Peter Junior, PJ. "I had to get up, I didn't have time to suffer, I had to take care of this boy. You told me that one day, if I lost weight, the blood pressure, cholesterol and diabetes, everything else would follow. I have this little kid, and he needs a man in his life. I took charge of what I could. I cleaned out my pantry, we signed up for supermarket online shopping, which was a blessing, not only for our health, but for our budget. We started eating mostly vegetables, fruits, nuts, mushrooms, beans, fish, and occasionally chicken. I hate counting calories, it takes the fun away from the joy of eating, but what surprised me was that I started feeling a burst of energy no later than a week after I made this change. I started walking, every day more and more. My sleep got better. I also put the sleep machine to use. Now I know what it means to have a full night of rest. I went back to my tools and started working in my wood shop. PJ loves to spend time with me in there. See the pictures of the armchairs I now make …"

Listening to Peter's health journey, looking at his radiant smile, I saw a man in charge who had joined forces with his body's self-healing powers. "I'm going to fight it!" Driven by a powerful purpose, he declared himself to be captain in this battle and used his own arsenal of mindful interventions to fight the longstanding lifestyle habits that had led him to overeating, under moving, and over reliance on medications. His illnesses or the misery of them eventually drove him to positive transformation.

We always have a choice—either succumb to the limitations and disabilities of the chronic illness or fight to maintain the part of our lives that brings joy and serves purpose.

Ask yourself, why do you want to wake up every morning? Why do you want to beat cancer? Why do you want to be able to … Find your purpose.

DISTORTED REALITY

We doubt that our brain can provide us with thoughts distorted from reality. "Who knows better than my own body?" We accept that people around us are diagnosed with cancer, but we think it won't happen to us. Surprise! Our brain is prone to biases that we don't think of. Do we perceive ourselves as being superior to the average human being? Yes, we commonly do. As researchers say, we experience "superiority illusions." We are confident that we won't have a heart attack, even if we consume pounds of fast food and spend every evening binging on TV shows instead of hitting the gym. We think we won't get COVID-19 and don't wear masks or get vaccinated. Even if we do, we're going to be fine. The *optimism bias* (discussed in Chapter 2) is a cognitive illusion. Human brains need positive biases to survive, to keep our minds at ease moving us forward despite fear.[348]

Psychosocial studies show that people overrate themselves by overestimating the likelihood that they will engage in desirable behaviors and achieve favorable outcomes.[349] College students think they're less likely to gain a drinking problem or suffer a heart attack.[350] We are unrealistically optimistic about our own health risks compared with those of other people.

People think they are less susceptible to the flu than their peers and, as a result, avoid getting flu shots.[351] Most of the time, we overestimate how healthy our behavior is. The statement, "I eat healthily, but still can't lose weight," quickly becomes hypothetical after we journal our actual food intake.

HELPLESSNESS IS OVERRATED

American psychologist Martin Seligman developed the theory of learned helplessness in the late '60s. In his experiments, when dogs were given painful shocks and could stop them by pressing a lever, they quickly learned to stop the pain. Dogs also figured out how to escape a kennel cage. The dogs who weren't given a way to stop the pain, learned to tolerate it. They lay down and cried in a kennel, even if the escape route was available. Seligman interpreted this concept into human behavior as when we feel we cannot control circumstances, we stop taking actions to eliminate the barriers.[352] You cannot control your genetics, but you can tackle the way you live with chronic illness.

Since the time when the learned helplessness theory came out, psychologists have figured out that passivity in response to shock is actually not learned. It is the default, unlearned response to prolonged aversive events. The suffering could be controlled and improved with behavior change.

"Being a patient, especially being a patient with a chronic condition, is a lot of work. And there's no curriculum about the work of being a patient," said Dr. Victor Montori, professor of medicine at the Mayo Clinic in Rochester, Minnesota.[353]

"Will I ever be *healthy?*" asked Harry, with sadness and hope at the same time. I love this question because it leads to a conversation about taking responsibility for your actions and helps to cultivate resilience from chronic illness' destructive course.

We live in a world where Western medicine, with its modern technological and pharmaceutical victories, firmly takes precedence. The Western approach assigns the primary emphasis to the individual's body and environment as only one factor that affects it. While medications, procedures and surgeries will treat cells, tissues, and organs, they will not return your body to the same status quo that it had before. In the process of treatment, which might be lifelong, you can either focus on the illness and the burden it brings, or painfully and intentionally choose a different life with illness "on board." There are a lot of historical figures who lived remarkable lives despite the burden of chronic illness.

Julius Caesar, for example, wouldn't have been able to defeat his political rival Pompey in a civil war and lead Rome until his assassination if he'd put all his energy into suffering from epilepsy and mini-strokes. Charles Darwin suffered from persistent vomiting, headaches, recurrent boils, panic attacks, and "hysterical crying and stroke-like episodes." Somehow, he made the greatest discovery of the theory of evolution by natural selection. Abraham Lincoln is thought to have had Marfan syndrome, which places challenges on connective tissue, affecting the skeleton, lungs, eyes, heart, and blood vessels. He also suffered from incapacitating depression. Winston Churchill, George Washington and Franklin D. Roosevelt all endured serious chronic medical conditions and lived public lives at the highest level, making historic decisions.[354] Those are just a few examples of how, through medical care, drive, purpose, and channeling effort, people can endure and win the battle with chronic illness toward vitality.

If we can't cure chronic illness, can we prolong vitality as part of healing? As in, not prolonging our lifespan, but having years of a rewarding, meaningful and happy life? There is plenty of research and scientific accomplishments that prove we can. Future breakthroughs are happening all the time as new transplants, medications, gene therapies, epigenetic programming, and many other fascinating things advance. I am excited about that future. But what could you do today to lessen the burden of chronic illnesses?

Healing accompanies the experience of transcending suffering, which results in harmony, wellbeing, balance, and peace. It's independent of restoration of function and recovery from or cure of disease. It therefore remains a viable option for chronically and terminally ill patients.[355] By refocusing from the illness to preserving personal integrity and restoring wellbeing, we can still heal, even with a chronic illness.

"What helped you to be successful and happy in your job?" I asked Harry. There were three powers that Harry told me about. He loved order and knew how to set up a habitual process for new interventions. He also thrived on taking charge. Most importantly, Harry had an optimistic outlook on life. Using these three powers, we came up with a list of actions:

- Accept responsibility for three behavior changes over time until they become a habit. It usually takes 60 days to build a habit: monitor blood pressure, decrease salt intake, and be physically active for 150 minutes a week.

- Instead of hiding symptoms of stress and exhaustion, acknowledge them, write them down together with the triggers.

- Stick to the medication regimen for six months to let the lifestyle changes take place.

One of the habits Harry struggled with in his job was trying to be perfect and allowing himself to spend long hours to achieve that goal. We included in the plan to be gentle with the body as a good friend, listen to its signs and give encouragement, when necessary, without pushing too hard.

Three months later, Harry had lost 5lb, his blood pressure was at goal. He was optimistic, proud of himself for visiting the gym three times a week and making dietary changes with the help of his wife. He reduced his salt intake and had cleaned out processed food from his pantry. Together with his wife, they explored new recipes for dishes using mostly plant-based foods. During his next yearly physical exam, Harry proudly acknowledged the 25lb weight loss he'd achieved and was feeling good. He and his wife both decided to become vegetarians. His cholesterol and blood sugar were at goal, and we decided to taper down his blood pressure medication.

The body has powers for self-healing. Acknowledging this fact doesn't mean stopping monitoring for symptoms or signs, quite the opposite. Take control of your body's healing process, try to not sabotage its efforts, and enhance self-healing by bringing in professional medical help. This is "real" healthcare.

CHECK YOUR HEALTHCARE INVENTORY:

1. Do you have any self-sabotaging habits that led or may lead you to chronic illness?

2. Is there anything you can and want to change? Set some achievable goals today.

CHAPTER 27

POWER TO HEAL

Seeing naked human beings is part of the daily practice in a doctor's office. "Please get undressed behind the curtain. Here is a gown for you and a sheet to cover yourself. When you're ready, let me know." That's how it goes. Not that morning.

"Hi, Kathy, how are you?" I stepped into the patient's room with a smile and an outstretched hand to see 51-year-old Kathy Huborg, my 8am patient, sitting naked on the chair next to the desk. She looked peaceful, with her hands circled around her protruding white belly with fingers locked below her exposed breasts. She unlocked them, stood up to greet me and shook my hand. "Hi, Doctor G."

While controlling my thoughts and emotions, my brain sometimes neglects to synchronize them with the expressions on my face. My face followed my real emotions instead of the commands of my brain. It took me a millisecond to consciously "make a face" appropriate for the situation. *Did Amanda [my medical assistant] forget to give Kathy a gown?* I wondered. The medical assistant helps patients to change into the gown in preparation for a physical exam. I saw the gown, stretched out on the exam table. After 20 years in healthcare and ten of them with me, Amanda does not forget. It was clear that Kathy didn't want to put the gown on. *Don't look surprised*, I commanded my face.

Kathy's clinic visit was scheduled to follow up her recent admission to hospital for atrial fibrillation, a condition where the heart trembles irregularly, often rapidly, leading to blood clot development in the heart. If a clot breaks off and gets into the bloodstream, it sticks to an artery in the brain, resulting in a stroke. Kathy was a frequent flier in our residents' and faculty daily medicine clinic. Atrial fibrillation was a recent illness that Kathy had to battle through in addition to her high blood pressure, sleep apnea, obesity, high cholesterol, and depression. Usually, Kathy was seen by one of our residents. We discussed Kathy frequently and, as the attending, I examined Kathy with residents to make sure the diagnosis and treatment were correct.

Kathy was also a Balint group patient. The Balint group are clinicians within the same office who meet regularly to present clinical cases in order to better understand the clinician-patient relationship. It's not about medical dilemmas, but about a patient's story and the role of a doctor. Being a Balint leader for decades had helped me to be open to the realization that I might be wrong about patients' perceptions and guided me toward developing more productive patient-doctor relationships. Kathy was a patient who challenged residents, being called a "difficult patient." Different residents kept bringing her case to discuss during group meetings from year to year. Despite using all the correct methods of treatments of her medical conditions, neither the doctors nor Kathy felt satisfied that all the right things were done medically. Kathy kept coming back looking for something that we were not able to give.

Today, Kathy was sitting naked, except for white socks and worn white tennis shoes, in the chair next to my desk. "Let me get Amanda, my medical assistant." I opened the door looking for a chaperone. Doctors like to use a chaperone to protect patients' privacy and respect patients' dignity during sensitive examinations. Amanda, with her years of wisdom from caring for thousands of patients, didn't wonder about the nakedness of our patient, she just pulled the blue gown off the exam table and handed it to Kathy. "I am fine," Kathy said, refusing to wear the gown. *We may have ten elephants in the room, but we also have atrial fibrillation to take care of*, I thought. That was familiar and easy. Let's focus on atrial fibrillation.

"Do you still have palpitations, Kathy? Do you feel tired? Any signs of bleeding? Let me listen to your heart and look at your legs. Any swelling? No? Great."

I adjusted her medications to control her heartrate and her dose of blood thinner. "You can get dressed, Kathy." She looked at me with deep sadness that made me feel like a coward for being scared to approach something important to her. I took a deep breath and stepped into less-comfortable territory. "What's going on, Kathy?"

I knew that patients may not express their needs in words. The real concerns must be discovered by the doctor's exploration and sometimes intuition. "To satisfy such a patient does not mean simply to satisfy the patient's expressed wishes, but to fulfill deeper, often unconscious, needs," wrote Philip Hopkins in the book *Patient Centered Medicine*.[356]

"I have been coming to this office for almost ten years," said Kathy. "I see doctors, good doctors. I take all medications. I don't feel good. My health is getting worse and worse. I'm here, do you 'see' me, can you tell me how to get back to normal?" In other words, Kathy was asking, "Can you heal me?"

Relieving suffering or healing is the ancient goal central to medicine's meaning and purpose.[357] "Heal" means "to make sound or whole" and comes from the root, *haelan*, the condition of being *hal*, whole.[358] *Hal* is also the root of "holy," defined as "spiritually pure." As early as 400 BC, Hippocrates described healing as a natural process leading to restoration of wholeness, creating harmony between body and soul.[359] Can medicine, with pills, surgeries, and devices, overturn the impact of illness on the body and spirit? As much as we want it to happen, repair of physical functions doesn't immediately restore emotional, social, psychological, and spiritual attributes. When patients desperately look for healing that represents body and mind, clinicians are focused on cure of diseases.

Within the 15–20 minutes of patients' encounters, clinicians can barely accomplish a plan of treatment and set it into action by placing orders, discussing them with patients and planning follow-ups. Cardiologists treat heart diseases, neurologists take care of diseases of nerves, gastroenterologists cure the gut. Who does the "whole body healing"? With the specialization of Western medicine, when different physicians take care of different body systems or diseases and don't see patients regularly, the ability to understand physical and spiritual needs becomes limited. If we accept the fact that medical science contributes to the diagnosis and treatment of illnesses, but doesn't engage in every aspect of human suffering and healing, what roles in the recovery from illness and returning to "normal" do doctors play? Are physicians prepared to take on the role of healers and relieve suffering when cure is the primary purpose of medicine? Some physicians question the legitimacy and their moral authority in the guidance of patients through healing journeys.

Why do patients ask doctors for advice when 70 to 80 percent of lifestyle advice is ignored?[360] Some 50 to 60 percent of long-term medications go unfinished, every third prescription for chronic health conditions are never filled, and about half are not taken as prescribed.[361] I am not surprised that physicians' advice has limited power. Healing from illness is our own intense, personal experience, where medicine plays an important, but specified, limited, advising role. It takes time to find meaning, balance, and acceptance in our experiences to heal.

WHY DOES THE DOCTOR'S ADVICE NOT WORK?

Researchers from the University of Washington conducted a study looking at what healing means to patients, physicians, and clinical staff. Surprisingly, all groups agreed on the definition of healing as a "multidimensional process of restoring a sense of wellbeing." A sense of wellbeing was defined by both patients and health professionals as a person's mental, spiritual, and physical health.[362] All groups acknowledged that "healing requires the person to reach a point of personal balance and acceptance" and, "relationships are essential to healing." Healing necessitates understanding the patient as a whole person, not just addressing medical problems. Doctors can diagnose, treat, and prevent diseases, but it's a human's capability to heal that determines the final outcome.

Chronic illness pushes people to change their behavior, which is one of the hardest things to do. No wonder that only 5 percent of the adult US population can maintain positive lifestyle behaviors.[363] Temporary changes in behavior are unlikely to have substantial effects on chronic illness. The challenge is not only to find a suitable intervention, but to be able to maintain it to continue healing.

What about the barriers to follow the physician's advice? The first barrier is based on the fact that up to half of patients have difficulty understanding what their doctor tells them about why they are sick and how to take the medications they are given.

The second reason clinicians' recommendations fail is a lack of patient trust that the advice is going to work. In the era of availability of information on the internet, many choose to disregard doctors' advice for reasons such as having read articles in the non-medical literature, making their own interpretation of medical research, or basing their decisions on what they've seen on television or heard from friends.

There is a much larger group of people who want to follow clinicians' recommendations but stop after a week or two for unknown reasons. Most of those are not cost related. They are the same for clinicians and patients. It's hard to take medications every day and not see immediate improvement. It takes time to exercise. It's not pleasant to eat healthy food if it doesn't bring joy. Changing longstanding habits is disruptive and the results might not be visible for months.

What about a physician's advice on nutrition or complementary medicine? In the US, 18.9 percent of adults had used at least one mind-body therapy within the last year, and every third adult plans to continue using alternative and complementary medicine.[364] "Talk to your doctor if this method is for you," patients hear in almost every complementary therapy advertisement. The truth is, as we mentioned earlier, doctors don't learn complementary and alternative therapies in allopathic medical schools. In a report published by the Harvard Food Law and Policy Clinic, researchers wrote that, on average, students in medical schools across the country spend less than one percent of lecture time learning about diet.[365]

Doctors learn biochemistry of proteins, sugars, and lipids, and consequences of poor lifestyle habits, but not how to teach self-care skills, secrets of food, and culinary medicine or exercise techniques. Some physicians justify this lack of knowledge and defer this task to psychologists or nutritionists, or they deny mind and body therapies entirely.

Some physicians call using natural remedies, alternative therapies or complementary medicine pseudoscience, closing their eyes to the fact that every second patient with chronic diseases and cancer uses CAM remedies together with their treatment. In surveys, 90 percent of Americans use and want to add mind and body therapies to their conventional care.[366]

"What else can I do to heal?" patients ask. I love that question because the alternative is that instead of getting professional advice, some people may delay treatments, start a new miracle diet or spend hundreds of dollars on a shiny supplement that promises a fountain of energy, pain relief, and forever happiness.

A Norwegian study on cancer patients suggested that positive communication experiences with their physicians led to CAM use as

a supplement rather than an alternative to conventional methods.[367]
Dutch studies have found that the patients who used their primary
care doctor's advice with complementary medicine training had lower
mortality rates and cost less to the healthcare system due to shorter
hospital stays and fewer drug prescriptions.[368]

My kudos to those patients who continue looking into other
options to heal. This is an acknowledgment of their personal responsibility in the healing journey.

CHECK YOUR HEALTHCARE INVENTORY:

1. Think through your personal achievements; can you identify
   three anchors that have helped you to succeed or survive?

2. How can you use these anchors against your health challenges?

CHAPTER 28

HEALING BODY AND MIND

We live in our body, sometimes without knowing and believing its capability to restore itself, thinking that all bodily functions are fragile. We look for a magic pill or genie in a bottle. What if you had the most powerful self-driving vehicle in your garage given to you for free? This is the only vehicle you could have forever. With all reasonable doubt, nobody can advise you for sure to what extent you can count on self-healing powers or your body's potential to overcome certain illnesses and maintain health. But there are general basics that we can count on. I won't push you into studying physiology, but learning your body, similar to how you learn a new vehicle, is the first step in answering this question. It takes time to discover its capabilities and reactions while you "actively" monitor "the drive" and seek help when it fails. Your body is a fascinating self-regulatory machine capable of natural repair and recovery of mind, body, and spirit.

Martha Sager was known to our practice as a frequent caller at night. At age 56, divorced, a chemist researcher, she lived alone and woke frequently with palpitations, or fast heartbeats. She underwent extensive cardiac evaluation, and her laboratory tests were completely normal. We also tested her for sleep apnea, but the test came back negative. Her PCP tried to start medications that could reduce her heartrate, called beta-blockers, but she felt tired during the daytime and refused to take them. After multiple evaluations in the ED, she refused to go there at all.

Our consensus was that she had an anxiety disorder. But the generalized anxiety surveys—instruments we use to diagnose patients with anxiety disorders—were also persistently negative. She also didn't want to try any medications, since "the anxiety test was negative." The problem was overwhelming not only for Martha, but for our physicians on call. Physicians in our practice knew her name and the lack of help they could provide during the night.

When I received the phone call at 2am, Martha was breathing fast and had her usual palpitations. I asked her to check her pulse, it was 105 (heartrate is normal between 60–100 bpm). Her blood pressure was normal. I asked Martha to breathe with me, counting every breath 1-2-3-4, and introduced her to the 4-7-8 breathing technique;[369] a slow breathing technique.[370] Research evidence suggests that *diaphragmatic breathing exercises* may help to reduce stress, based not only on mental health self-evaluations, but on cortisol levels and blood pressure measurements. Controlled, slow breathing appears to be an effective means of maximizing heartrate variability (HRV) and preserving autonomic function (the major system participating in the stress reaction), both of which have been associated with decreased mortality in pathological states and longevity.[371]

After three cycles of 4-7-8 breathing, Martha's heartrate reduced to 80 and she felt much relieved. The following day we saw her in the office and confirmed again that her electrocardiogram continued to be normal. We agreed that she would do at least four exercises with 4-7-8 breathing before going to sleep and as soon as she woke at night. That ended her night calls. Three months later, Martha told me that this "magic breathing cured her palpitations."

What is most fascinating is that slow breathing, as mindfulness, is always available when you're stressed, anxious and waiting for a procedure, and in many other situations when you want to achieve calmness.

Hopefully, at some point there will be studies to prove the benefits of mind and body techniques at the DNA level. It doesn't mean we should discard the benefits of influencing the mind on healing. If stress can cause harm, which has been proven in many research studies, safe interventions that cause relaxation can and should be used by individuals who believe in them to enhance self-healing. When remedies can help and have been helping many for centuries, is it wise to disregard them? I don't think so.

Mind and body techniques connect subconscious emotional thoughts and behaviors with physical health. They trigger the relaxation response that helps with stress reduction and healing. Laughter can stimulate circulation, soothe tension, and increase endorphins released by the brain. Religious practices and the power of prayer have been associated with healing for millennia. How do they participate in the healing process? Using pliability of the brain—attributable to the process called neuroplasticity—mind and body therapies reduce reactivity to the fight–flight–freeze reaction that is initiated in response to perceived danger. By learning techniques and creating habits of using them, we also count on neuroplasticity of the brain to enhance healing.

In the late 19th century, Josef Breuer, an Austrian physician and physiologist, discovered that one of his patients, Anna O—a young woman suffering from hysteria and temporary paralysis—could be cured through hypnosis. She couldn't speak her native German but could speak French and English and couldn't drink water even when thirsty. Breuer discovered that if he hypnotized her, she would talk about things she didn't remember while being in a conscious state, and afterwards her symptoms were relieved; thus, it was called "the talking cure." This discovery gave Sigmund Freud, an Austro-Hungarian physician, the idea of psychoanalysis, recognizing the possibility of controlling the unconscious mind and influencing the way people feel.

I understand people's skepticism. I was a skeptic too when I showed up for a hypnosis lecture as a medical student, which was given to us by one of the traveling professors from Saint Petersburg. Young and fashionably dressed, Dr. Korolenko didn't look like a professor who'd published books and hundreds of medical articles. I was sitting in the back row with a group of students who saw themselves mostly in the surgical specialties and had come there just to get the credit. We all smiled when the professor asked us to interlace our fingers, but we followed his command. After he spoke a few more sentences, I started feeling tightness close to pain in my fingers. The strangest thing happened—I couldn't free up my fingers from being locked.

The pain was getting stronger, and my fingers became a bluish color. My smile changed to fear. Relief came when Dr. Korolenko asked students with "locked" fingers to come to the stage. Usually, you couldn't make me go to the stage for any reason. In fact, I'd missed most of the award ceremonies just to avoid getting on stage. Looking at my bluish fingers made me run to the stage with a group of others with the same tightly locked-up fingers. I remember every word the professor said on stage, "Close your eyes, breathe deeply, in and out. Feel the sun shining on your face. Open your arms to the sun." I couldn't resist turning my head to the imagined sun and raising my hands, which immediately unlocked. He was talking about feeling strong and powerful, getting energy from the sun.

I didn't have a smile after this lecture. It was time for spring break, but I, for unknown reasons, spent days studying German from books and tapes, which was absolutely useless for my medical school learning, instead of having a good time with my friends. I felt an incredible amount of energy too, which made me believe in the power of the mind.

Would you say that your body is capable of literally shaking off stress and even mental trauma? Remember yourself as a child being scared walking through a dark alley somewhere, and your body started shaking? Many people shake after a motor vehicle accident, even when they aren't injured. We try to stop the shaking because we don't know that it's something the body does to release stress. It's an involuntary, healthy, self-healing mechanism that has been used by Dr. David Berceli to create TRE (tension and trauma release exercises).[372] By using a similar but self-induced tremor to mechanically discharge physical tension, TRE thereby releases the experience of excess stress.[373] For 22 years, Berceli lived and worked in war-torn countries of Africa and the Middle East, providing trauma recovery assistance to US military personnel of national and international organizations whose staff were living and working in trauma-induced environments. I didn't believe that shaking or tremor could be controlled until I attended Dr. Berceli's teaching session for myself.

More than 50 physicians were lying on their backs on the floor with their knees bent and the soles of their feet pressed together in the "butterfly pose," as this traditional hip-opener position is called in yoga. Dr. Berceli asked us to pick our pelvis up off the ground with open knees. By slowly closing the knees, we found ourselves shaking, more or less. The mechanism of induced shaking comes from activation of the adductor muscles that are in the inner thighs of the leg. The tremors sustain themselves, which was a big surprise to the field of physiology. I was skeptical until the moment my body started convulsing in small shaking movements, which stopped immediately when I got out of the suggested pose.

"For people who are doing this for the first time," said Dr. Berceli, "if you just have stress or tension, these are kind of innocent, and you can do them easily and you don't have a problem. But if you're going to be working with some trauma or certainly a developed mental trauma that has a lot of psycho-emotional stuff attached to it, you may want to do this with a certified TRE practitioner."[374] This is one of the mind and body therapies that is based on the same principle that the body uses for self-healing: releasing stress through shaking.

Mind and body practices, such as acupuncture, massage therapy, meditation, mindful eating, relaxation techniques, tai chi, and yoga have good safety records and can be added to conventional methods when done properly and taught by trained and qualified professionals. Chronic medical conditions or other special circumstances (such as pregnancy, cancer or severe PTSD) may affect the safety of mind and body practices and so should be addressed with your physician prior to considering any of them.

As with any healing technique, mind and body therapies may also exacerbate symptoms of chronic health conditions, especially mental illness. Patients complain of hip, neck, and shoulder pain from overuse injuries during yoga sessions or falls from losing balance during tai chi. When added to traditional treatments, there might be unpredictable reactions, thoughts and emotions that may influence anxiety outcomes. You have to find the right fit; a practitioner can advise you about using the techniques in small increments, paying attention to the reactions of the body. There is an old saying, "Pain is a teacher." If you feel pain or discomfort after a body movement, stop and try to analyze what's happened and ask for advice.

Chronic illness rarely comes alone, and treatments bring new challenges, making twists and turns on the way toward vitality, but if you're diagnosed with an illness, consider your health as a pivot point: accept the current stage of your health and deal with its positives and negatives. You can sway the direction it goes. Focus on your health today and work on strategies to enhance the body's self-healing process, instead of focusing on the illness. Let doctors find the best treatment options for your illness.

The Eastern idea of health and disease is perceived as two sides of a coin. It considers every individual being in a state of balance between external insults and internal defensive mechanisms. For example, traditional Chinese medicine teaches that the human body changes through a cycle of "becoming, releasing, transforming, dying, and rebirth." As we know, the environment that the body tries to adapt to varies for every individual and is based on longstanding habits. People's bodies adapt to external changes to live in balance within themselves and their environment, thereby maintaining good health. If the insults are greater than your defenses, you become ill; if not, you maintain good health.[375] Adaptation to the changing environment during long-lasting illness affects the body and the mind. Eastern medicine relies on the bond between the mind, body, and spirit to bring balance to a person's spiritual, emotional, mental, and physical health.

My doubts about the exclusive powers of the Western approach to treat chronic illnesses led me to stop repeatedly asking my patients to "eat healthily and exercise." It's hard, not all people can make lifelong sacrifices. Instead, I use my limited time with patients to discover each individual's motivator that would lead them towards recovery and better health. Knowing those, which are different for everyone, will help to open the door toward hope that another change is possible.

I GOT THIS!

It is not a secret that if you believe in the power of medication or a procedure, the outcome might be more favorable. This response is called the placebo effect. Placebo response is also an example of mind and body connection during healing that usually involves the mind, body, and spirit.

The word placebo comes from the Latin phrase "I shall please."[376] Placebos were present in Ancient Rome and Greece, the Bible, Renaissance Europe in the forms of chants, potions, boiled dung, lizard blood, mold and unicorn horn, incubation in a temple or touch… you name it.

In 1772, William Cullen demonstrably used the term placebo for the first time in his lectures "to fulfill the patient's desire for a remedy even though he did not personally believe in its pharmacological effectiveness."[377] Can we count on the placebo effect? I would count on anything if it's harmless and easy to deliver.

We as clinicians use the placebo effect many times a day. When clinicians prescribe new medication, they use the psychological power of the placebo effect by saying, "This medication *will* resolve your symptoms." Most likely it will. But it also could give potentially dangerous side effects, which we are aware of, but hope will not happen. When physicians support prescribing medication with a positive message, patients are more likely to also believe in the effect and are more likely to refill the prescription and take it as prescribed. If we start with the description of the side effect, we use the *nocebo effect*— the opposite of the placebo—negative reinforcement. Negative messages about the medication influence patients to stop it.

We want to count on the placebo effect of positive affirmations in our healing. "I am strong, I got this!" or "This is going to work!" or "My hair is falling out, the chemotherapy is working!" or "My body is healing, I am grateful." Self-affirmation is a practice of thinking or writing about your core values. A large body of psychology studies have shown that self-affirmations help buffer a variety of stressors, including chronic illness, stress and rumination associated with the fear of death. The link between ventromedial prefrontal cortex (VMPFC) activity during health message exposure and behavior change may stem from the recipient's ability to process a health message as self-relevant or as having value to oneself.

Emily B. Falk, PhD, with researchers from the University of Pennsylvania, University of Michigan, Ann Arbor, and University of California, used functional magnetic resonance imaging (fMRI) to examine neural processes associated with affirmation effects during exposure to potentially threatening health messages in the ventromedial prefrontal cortex (VMPFC), a brain region selected for its association with self-related processing and positive valuation. More importantly, they proved that the brain changes from self-affirmations led to objective behavior change.[378]

However, as a big promoter of positive thinking, I also know that repeating motivational statements does not work for everyone. Dr. Joanne Wood, with Canadian researchers at the University of Waterloo, showed that they can backfire for people with low self-esteem, or at times when self-esteem needs a boost, which is frequently the case for those with chronic illnesses. They found that for those with low self-esteem, positive affirmations triggered a negative feeling of being "not good enough." Instead, they found a better mood when "allowed to have negative thoughts about themselves" and asking questions "how do I get better?" By introducing neutral reality-based statements, such as "I am not great, but I will be. I am okay," we line up the path towards believing and accepting that one day "I got this!"[379]

My initial reaction to my "broken heart" syndrome that could potentially kill me was fear mixed with disappointment. *What bad luck!* I thought. *Why did God not send me a "normal" coronary artery disease? A disease that has known treatments with explored outcomes. I could get a stent placed in one of my coronary arteries or even go through a coronary artery bypass. Many of my patients have had excellent outcomes after surgical interventions and lifestyle changes.* I questioned my beliefs in following healthy lifestyle habits, which I religiously practiced, and in the medications I'd prescribed for decades. I even started feeling petty about myself and my future. Until, one day, my adult son showed up on my doorstep.

He was just 11 years old when, together with his little sister, I pulled them from our extended family roots in Russia and planted new roots in the United States. As any teenager from an immigrant family, he'd had his own life challenges to go through. My boy flew from another part of the world, where he worked at that time, to tell me, "Get up, Mama. Get up, let's go!" Words that I used to tell him quite frequently, years ago. Why did I believe him, instead of my own medical knowledge and experience? Maybe because he, more than anyone, was aware of our Siberian resilient roots and knew that I had to be the one to get me out of the "illness" mode and into the "well" mode.

We started walking, first around the neighborhood, then close by parks, every day increasing the distance and speed. We didn't talk about diseases or medications, mostly concentrating on our past life in Siberia, other people who'd had to go through challenges and not only survived but thrived after. It was nothing magical. Learning new things, believing in myself and my body, having a purpose and looking for a community of people who'd overcome or known how to overcome similar misfortunes. My new knowledge of integrative medicine had found the right soil for the scientific explanations of ancient remedies of Eastern medicine that I grew up with. I wasn't intimidated anymore by modern technologies and medical successes of Western medicine. Instead, I was ready to combine the wisdom of both, becoming my own integrative medicine patient. The trembling bird, which had made a nest in my "broken heart" at some point vanished, leaving me with another life lesson of self-reliance and commonsense.

CHECK YOUR HEALTHCARE INVENTORY:

1. What are your biggest motivators?

2. Make a mental list of people, including doctors, you would reach out to for medical advice? Is there anyone else you would like to have on your "Board of Advisors"? Search for them and reach out to them.

ONLINE RESOURCES

Agency for Healthcare Research and Quality (AHRQ)

https://www.ahrq.gov/

20 Tips to Help Prevent Medical Errors: Patient Fact Sheet
https://www.ahrq.gov/questions/resources/20-tips.html#:~:text=
The%20best%20way%20you%20can,tend%20to%20get%20better
%20results.

Personal Health Literacy Measurement Tools
https://www.ahrq.gov/health-literacy/research/tools/index.html
#short

Centers for Disease Control and Prevention

https://www.cdc.gov/

Adult BMI Calculator
https://www.cdc.gov/healthyweight/assessing/bmi/adult_bmi/
english_bmi_calculator/bmi_calculator.html

Assessing Your Weight
https://www.cdc.gov/healthyweight/assessing/index.html

Choosing Wisely ®

https://www.choosingwisely.org/patient-resources/

Cleveland Clinic

https://my.clevelandclinic.org/

Breast Self-Exam
https://my.clevelandclinic.org/health/diagnostics/3990-breast
-self-exam

Cochrane Library

https://www.cochranelibrary.com/

Cochrane Database of Systematic Reviews
https://www.cochranelibrary.com/cdsr/about-cdsr

ConsumerLab.com

https://www.consumerlab.com/

Consumer Reports

Have a Better Hospital Stay
https://www.consumerreports.org/hospitals/have-a-better-hospital
-stay-how-to-handle-inpatient-issues/

DPC Mapper

https://mapper.dpcfrontier.com/

Familydoctor.org

https://familydoctor.org/

The American Geriatrics Society's (AGS)

https://geriatricscareonline.org/

Google Scholar

https://scholar.google.com/

Health On the Net

https://hon.ch/en/

Tools
https://www.hon.ch/en/tools.html

Healthline

https://www.healthline.com/

John Hopkins Medicine

https://www.hopkinsmedicine.org/

Vital signs
https://www.hopkinsmedicine.org/health/conditions-and-diseases/
vital-signs-body-temperature-pulse-rate-respiration-rate-blood-
pressure

Leapfrog Hospital Safety Grade

https://www.hospitalsafetygrade.org/

Medicare

https://www.medicare.gov/

Find & compare providers near you
https://www.medicare.gov/care-compare/?providerType=Hospital
&redirect=true

MedlinePlus

https://www.medlineplus.gov/

Mayo Clinic

https://www.mayoclinic.org/

Testicular exam

https://www.mayoclinic.org/tests-procedures/testicular-exam/about/pac-20385252

National Cancer Institute (NCI)

https://www.cancer.gov/

Lunch Cancer Screening

https://www.cancer.gov/types/lung/patient/lung-screening-pdq

Skin Cancer Screening

https://www.cancer.gov/types/skin/patient/skin-screening-pdq

National Center for Complementary and Integrative Health

https://www.nccih.nih.gov/

National Institutes of Health (NIH)

https://www.nih.gov/

Dietary Supplement Fact Sheets

https://ods.od.nih.gov/factsheets/list-all/

National Library of Medicine

https://www.nlm.nih.gov/

PubMed ®

https://pubmed.ncbi.nlm.nih.gov/

How to find information about complementary and integrative health practices on PubMed®

https://www.nccih.nih.gov/health/how-to-find-information-about-complementary-health-approaches-on-pubmed

Quality Check

https://www.qualitycheck.org/

U.S. Food & Drug Administration (FDA)

https://www.fda.gov/

Current Good Manufacturing Practice (CGMP) Regulations
https://www.fda.gov/drugs/pharmaceutical-quality-resources/
current-good-manufacturing-practice-cgmp-regulations

Dietary Supplement Products and Ingredients
https://www.fda.gov/food/dietary-supplements/dietary-supplement
-products-ingredients

U.S. Preventive Services Task Force

https://www.uspreventiveservicestaskforce.org/uspstf/

Risks associated with age and gender
https://www.uspreventiveservicestaskforce.org/uspstf/recommendation
-topics/uspstf-a-and-b-recommendations

WebMD

https://www.webmd.com/

NOTES

INTRODUCTION

1. Dias, Andre, Ivan J. Núñez Gil, Francesco Santoro, John E. Madias, Francesco Pelliccia, Natale Daniele Brunetti, Elena Salmoirago-Blotcher, Scott W. Sharkey et al. 2019, Jan. 1. "Takotsubo Syndrome: State-of-the-Art Review by an Expert Panel – Part 1." *Cardiovascular Revascularization Medicine* 20, no. 1: 70–9. https://doi.org/10.1016/j.carrev.2018.11.015.

2. Ryan, T. J., and J. T. Fallon. 1986. A 44-year-old woman with substernal pain and pulmonary edema after severe emotional stress. "Case Records of the Massachusetts General Hospital. Weekly Clinicopathological Exercises". Case 18. *New England Journal of Medicine* 314, no. 19: 1240–7.

3. Salleh, Mohd Razali. 2008. "Life Event, Stress and Illness." *Malaysian Journal of Medical Sciences* 15, no. 4: 9–18.

4. Citro, Rodolfo, Ilaria Radano, Guido Parodi, Davide Di Vece, Concetta Zito, Giuseppina Novo, Gennaro Provenza, Michele Bellino, Costantina Prota, Angelo Silverio, et al. 2019. "Long-Term Outcome in Patients with Takotsubo Syndrome Presenting with Severely Reduced Left Ventricular Ejection Fraction." *European Journal of Heart Failure* 21, no. 6: 781–9. https://doi.org/10.1002/ejhf.1373.

5. Medina de Chazal, Horacio, Marco Giuseppe Del Buono, Lori Keyser-Marcus, Liangsuo Ma, F. Gerard Moeller, Daniel Berrocal, and Antonio Abbate. 2018. "Stress Cardiomyopathy Diagnosis and Treatment: JACC State-of-the-Art Review." *Journal of the American College of Cardiology*, . 2018, October 16 72, no. 16: 1955–71. https://doi.org/10.1016/j.jacc.2018.07.072.

6. Dias, Andre, Ivan J. Núñez Gil, Francesco Santoro, John E. Madias, Francesco Pelliccia, Natale Daniele Brunetti, Elena Salmoirago-Blotcher, Scott W. Sharkey et al. 2019, Jan. 1. "Takotsubo Syndrome: State-of-the-Art Review by an Expert Panel – Part 1."

CHAPTER 1. DO YOUR PART

7. Roberts, Kathleen Johnston. 1999. "Patient Empowerment in the United States: a Critical Commentary." *Health Expectations: an International Journal of Public Participation in Health Care & Health Policy* 2, no. 2: 82–92. https://doi.org/10.1046/j.1369-6513.1999.00048.x.

8. The History of "Doctor" | Merriam-Webster. Accessed November 28, 2022. https://www.merriam-webster.com/words-at-play/the-history-of-doctor

9.   Neuberger, J., and R. Tallis. 1999. "Do We Need a New Word for Patients? Lets Do Away with "Patients"." *BMJ* 318, no. 7200: 1756–7. https://doi.org/10.1136/bmj.318.7200.1756.

CHAPTER 2. RISKS AND HEALTH MAP

10. Risk Definition & Meaning – Merriam-Webster. Accessed June 14, 2022. https://www.merriam-webster.com/dictionary/risk

11. Verweij, M. 2000. "What Is Preventive Medicine?" In *Canadian Family Physician* 20: 13–23.

12. A and B Recommendations | United States Preventive Services Taskforce. Accessed November 28, 2022. https://www.uspreventiveservicestaskforce.org/uspstf/recommendation-topics/uspstf-a-and-b-recommendations

13. [13] Kimura-Hayama, Eric T., Jesús A. Higuera, Roberto Corona-Cedillo, Laura Chávez-Macías, Anamari Perochena, Laura Yadira Quiroz-Rojas, Jesús Rodríguez-Carbajal, and José L. Criales. 2010. "Neurocysticercosis: Radiologic-Pathologic Correlation." *RadioGraphics* 30, no. 6: 1705–19. https://doi.org/10.1148/rg.306105522.

14. Valley Fever (Coccidioidomycosis) | Types of Fungal Diseases | Fungal | CDC. Accessed November 7, 2022. https://www.cdc.gov/fungal/diseases/coccidioidomycosis/index.html

15. Scurr, J. H., S. J. Machin, S. Bailey-King, I. J. Mackie, S. McDonald, and P. D. C. Smith. 2001. "Frequency and Prevention of Symptomless Deep-Vein Thrombosis in Long-Haul Flights: a Randomized Trial." *Lancet* 357, no. 9267: 1485–9. https://doi.org/10.1016/S0140-6736(00)04645-6

16. Pidgeon, N., C. Hood, D. Jones, B. Turner, and R. Gibson. 1992. "Risk Perception." In *Risk: Analysis, Perception and Management*, edited by Royal Society: 89–134. London: Royal Society.

17. Weinstein, N. D. 1980. "Unrealistic Optimism About Future Life Events." *Journal of Personality & Social Psychology* 39, no. 5: 806–20. https://doi.org/10.1037/0022-3514.39.5.806.

18. Sharot, T. 2012. *The Optimism Bias: A Tour of the Irrationally Positive Brain*. Vintage Book Company.

19. Alaszewski, Andy, and Tom Horlick-Jones. 2003. "How Can Doctors Communicate Information About Risk More Effectively?." *BMJ* 327, no. 7417: 728–31. https://doi.org/10.1136/bmj.327.7417.728.

20. Calman, K. C., P. G. Bennett, and D. G. Corns. 1999. "Risks to Health: Some Key Issues in Management, Regulation and Communication." *Health, Risk & Society* 1, no. 1: 107–16. https://doi.org/10.1080/13698579908407010.

CHAPTER 3. GENETIC LOAD

21. Phillips, Kathryn A., Patricia A. Deverka, Gillian W. Hooker, and Michael P. Douglas. 2018. "Genetic Test Availability and Spending: Where Are We Now? Where Are We Going?." *Health Affairs* 37, no. 5: 710–6. https://doi.org/10.1377/hlthaff.2017.1427.

22. Miller, N. H., V. L. Katz, and R. C. Cefalo. 1989. "Pregnancies Among Physicians. A Historical Cohort Study." *Journal of Reproductive Medicine* 34, no. 10: 790–6.

23. Carmeli, Daphna Birenbaum. 2004. "Prevalence of Jews as Subjects in Genetic Research: Figures, Explanation, and Potential Implications." *American Journal of Medical Genetics. Part A* 130A, no. 1: 76–83. https://doi.org/10.1002/ajmg.a.20291.

24. Gross, Susan J., Beth A. Pletcher, Kristin G. Monaghan, and Professional Practice and Guidelines Committee. 2008, Jan. "Carrier Screening in Individuals of Ashkenazi Jewish Descent." *Genetics in Medicine* 10, no. 1: 54–6. https://doi.org/10.1097/GIM.0b013e31815f247c.

25. Night, J. A., L. Jackson-Gusby, and W. White-Ryan. 2009. "Salem Health." *Cancer*. Pasadena, CA: Salem Press.

26. Phillips, K. A., Deverka, P. A., Hooker, G. W., & Douglas, M. P. 2018. "Genetic Test Availability and Spending: Where Are We Now? Where Are We Going?." *Health Affairs* 37, no. 5: 710–6. https://doi.org/10.1377/hlthaff.2017.1427.

27. "Our Health + Ancestry DNA Service 23andMe." Accessed March 7, 2021. https://www.23andme.com/dna-health-ancestry/?sub=ver2&cabt=nao

28. "23andMe for Medical Professionals – Understanding Personal Genetics." Accessed September 23, 2022. https://medical.23andme.com/

29. Oh, Bermseok. 2019. "Direct-to-Consumer Genetic Testing: Advantages and Pitfalls." *Genomics & Informatics* 17, no. 3: e33. https://doi.org/10.5808/GI.2019.17.3.e33.

30. Phillips, K. A., Deverka, P. A., Hooker, G. W., & Douglas, M. P. 2018. "Genetic Test Availability and Spending: Where Are We Now? Where Are We Going?." *Health Affairs* 37, no. 5: 710–6. https://doi.org/10.1377/hlthaff.2017.1427.

31. "Free Review of Ancestry DNA Tests | Genetics Digest." Accessed March 8, 2021. https://geneticsdigest.com/best_ancestry_genealogy_dna_test/index.html

32. "A consumer DNA testing company has given the FBI access to its two million profiles" | *MIT's Technology Review*. AccessedNovember 7, 2022. https://www.technologyreview.com/2019/02/01/137608/a-consumer-dna-testing-company-has-given-the-fbi-access-to-its-two-million/

CHAPTER 5. DROWNING IN INFORMATION

33. Battineni, Gopi, Simone Baldoni, Nalini Chintalapudi, Getu Gamo Sagaro, Graziano Pallotta, Giulio Nittari, and Francesco Amenta. 2020. "Factors Affecting the Quality and Reliability of Online Health Information." *Digital Health* 6: 2055207620948996. https://doi.org/10.1177/2055207620948996.

34. Lee, Kenneth, Kreshnik Hoti, Jeffery David Hughes, and Lynne Emmerton. 2014. "Dr Google and the Consumer: A Qualitative Study Exploring the Navigational Needs and Online Health Information-Seeking Behaviors of Consumers with Chronic Health Conditions." *Journal of Medical Internet Research* 16, no. 12: e262. https://doi.org/10.2196/jmir.3706.

35. Caiata-Zufferey, Maria, Andrea Abraham, Kathrin Sommerhalder, and Peter J. Schulz. 2010 Aug. "Online Health Information Seeking in the Context of the Medical Consultation in Switzerland." *Qualitative Health Research* 20, no. 8: 1050–61. https://doi.org/10.1177/1049732310368404.

36. Attfield, Simon J., Anne Adams, and Ann Blandford. 2006 Jun. "Patient Information Needs: Pre- and Post-consultation." *Health Informatics Journal* 12, no. 2: 165–77. https://doi.org/10.1177/1460458206063811.

37. Caiata-Zufferey, M., Abraham, A., Sommerhalder, K., Schulz, P. J. 2010 Aug. "Online Health Information Seeking in the Context of the Medical Consultation in Switzerland." *Qualitative Health Research* 20, no. 8: 1050–61. https://doi.org/10.1177/1049732310368404.

38. Rozmovits, Linda, and Sue Ziebland. 2004 Apr. "What Do Patients with Prostate or Breast Cancer Want from an Internet Site? A Qualitative Study of Information Needs.". *Patient Education & Counseling*. patient ed. 53, no. 1: 57–64. https://doi.org/10.1016/S0738-3991(03)00116-2.

39. Tustin, Nupur. 2010 Jan. "The Role of Patient Satisfaction in Online Health Information Seeking." *Journal of Health Communication* 15, no. 1: 3–17. https://doi.org/10.1080/10810730903465491.

40. LaValley, Susan A., Marc T. Kiviniemi, and Elizabeth A. Gage-Bouchard. 2017. "Where

People Look for Online Health Information." *Health Information & Libraries Journal* 34, no. 2: 146–55. https://doi.org/10.1111/hir.12143.

41. Semigran, Hannah L., Jeffrey A. Linder, Courtney Gidengil, and Ateev Mehrotra. 2015. "Evaluation of Symptom Checkers for Self-Diagnosis and Triage: Audit Study." *BMJ* 351: h3480. https://doi.org/10.1136/bmj.h3480.

42. "Online Health Information: Is It Reliable?", Accessed April 21, 2021 https://www.nia.nih.gov/health/online-health-information-it-reliable#where. National Institute on Aging.

43. "Weight-Loss Diet – Google Search". Google, Accessed September 25, 2022. https://www.google.com/search?q=weight-loss+diet&rlz=1C5CHFA_enUS694US696&oq=weight-loss+diet&aqs=chrome..69i57j69i65.627j0j4&sourceid=chrome&ie=UTF-8

44. "HONselect." *English* [Introduction], Accessed April 24, 2021. https://www.hon.ch/HONselect/index.html

45. "Tools and activities of the HON Foundation", Accessed April 24, 2021. https://www.hon.ch/20-years/en/tools.html#honcodeextension

CHAPTER 6. DECEPTION OF SELF-DIAGNOSIS

46. Fox, S., and M. Duggan. 2013. *Health Online 2013. Internet and American Life Project. Pew Research Center and California Health Care Foundation* vol. 4.

47. North, Frederick, William J. Ward, Prathibha Varkey, and Sidna M. Tulledge-Scheitel. 2012. "Should You Search the Internet for Information About Your Acute Symptom?." *Telemedicine Journal & e-Health* 18, no. 3: 213–8. https://doi.org/10.1089/tmj.2011.0127.

48. North, Frederick, William J. Ward, Prathibha Varkey, and Sidna M. Tulledge-Scheitel. 2012. "Should You Search the Internet for Information About Your Acute Symptom?." *Telemedicine Journal & e-Health* 18, no. 3: 213–8. https://doi.org/10.1089/tmj.2011.0127.

49. Kang, Cheol In, Jieun Kim, Dae Won Park, Baek Nam Kim, U. Syn Ha, Seung Ju Lee, Jeong Kyun Yeo, Seung Ki Min, Heeyoung Lee, and Seong Heon Wie. 2018. "Clinical Practice Guidelines for the Antibiotic Treatment of Community-Acquired Urinary Tract Infections." *Infection & Chemotherapy* 50, no. 1: 67–100. https://doi.org/10.3947/ic.2018.50.1.67.

50. Gawdat, M. 2017. *Solve for Happy: Engineer Your Path to Joy.* Gallery Press.

51. "Health Information Is a Popular Pursuit Online", Accessed January 18, 2022. https://www.pewresearch.org/internet/2011/02/01/health-information-is-a-popular-pursuit-online/. Pew Research Center.

CHAPTER 7. DECEIVING PERCEPTIONS

52. Prasad, N. R. 2021. "Perception and Reality." In *Studies in Computational Intelligence*, edited by A. Tversky, and D. Kahneman Rational choice and the framing of decisions. J. Bus 1986;59, 251–278 892: 193–218. https://doi.org/10.1086/296365.

53. Tversky, A., and D. Kahneman. 1986. "Rational Choice and the Framing of Decisions." *Journal of Business* 59, no. S4: 251–78. https://doi.org/10.1086/296365.

54. Kiefe, C. I., E. Funkhouser, M. N. Fouad, and D. S. May. 1998. "Chronic Disease as a Barrier to Breast and Cervical Cancer Screening." *Journal of General Internal Medicine* 13, no. 6: 357–65. https://doi.org/10.1046/j.1525-1497.1998.00115.x.

55. Ferrer, Rebecca A., William M. P. Klein, Aya Avishai, Katelyn Jones, Megan Villegas, and Paschal Sheeran. 2018. "When Does Risk Perception Predict Protection Motivation for

Health Threats? A Person-by-Situation Analysis." *PLOS ONE* 13, no. 3: e0191994. https://doi.org/10.1371/journal.pone.0191994.

56. Starcevic, Vladan, and David Berle. 2013, Feb. "Cyberchondria: Towards a Better Understanding of Excessive Health-Related Internet Use." *Expert Review of Neurotherapeutics* 13, no. 2: 205–13. https://doi.org/10.1586/ern.12.162.

57. Institute of Medicine. 2004. *Health Literacy: A Prescription to End Confusion Washington DC.* National Academies.

58. Davis, Terry C., and Michael S. Wolf. 2004. "Health Literacy: Implications for Family Medicine." *Family Medicine* 36, no. 8: 595–8.

59. "What Is Health Literacy? | Health Literacy." *CDC*, Accessed June 30, 2022. https://www.cdc.gov/healthliteracy/learn/index.html.

60. Hamm, R. M., and S. L. Smith. 1998. "The Accuracy of Patients' Judgments of Disease Probability and Test Sensitivity and Specificity." *Journal of Family Practice* 47, no. 1: 44–52.

61. Graham, Ian D., J. Logan, Margaret B. Harrison, Sharon E. Straus, Jacqueline Tetroe, Wenda Caswell, and Nicole Robinson. 2006. "Lost in Knowledge Translation: Time for a Map?." *Journal of Continuing Education in the Health Professions* 26, no. 1: 13–24. https://doi.org/10.1002/chp.47.

CHAPTER 8. TELL YOUR STORY

62. Peterson, M. C., J. H. Holbrook, D. Von Hales, N. L. Smith, and L. V. Staker. 1992. "Contributions of the History, Physical Examination, and Laboratory Investigation in Making Medical Diagnoses." *Western Journal of Medicine* 156, no. 2: 163–5. https://doi.org/10.1097/00006254-199210000-00013.

63. Lown B. 1999. *The Lost Art of Healing: Practicing Compassion in Medicine.* New York: Ballantine Books.

64. Levy, Andrea Gurmankin, Aaron M. Scherer, Brian J. Zikmund-Fisher, Knoll Larkin, Geoffrey D. Barnes, and Angela Fagerlin. 2018. "Prevalence of and Factors Associated with Patient Nondisclosure of Medically Relevant Information to Clinicians." *JAMA Network Open* 1, no. 7: e185293. https://doi.org/10.1001/jamanetworkopen.2018.5293.

65. "DASH Eating Plan." *NHLBI, NIH*, Accessed September 17, 2022. https://www.nhlbi.nih.gov/education/dash-eating-plan.

66. "Adult BMI Calculator | Healthy Weight, Nutrition, and Physical Activity." *CDC*, Accessed December 29, 2021. https://www.cdc.gov/healthyweight/assessing/bmi/adult_bmi/english_bmi_calculator/bmi_calculator.html.

67. Roter, D. 2000. "The Enduring and Evolving Nature of the Patient–Physician Relationship.". *Patient Education & Counseling*. patient ed. 39, no. 1: 5–15. https://doi.org/10.1016/s0738-3991(99)00086-5.

68. Hall, Judith A., Erik J. Coats, and Lavonia Smith LeBeau. 2005 Nov. "Nonverbal Behavior and the Vertical Dimension of Social Relations: A Meta-analysis." *Psychological Bulletin* 131, no. 6: 898–924. https://doi.org/10.1037/0033-2909.131.6.898.

CHAPTER 9. COMMUNICATION DANCE

69. Roter, D. 2000. "The Enduring and Evolving Nature of the Patient–Physician Relationship.". *Patient Education & Counseling*. patient ed. 39, no. 1: 5–15. https://doi.org/10.1016/s0738-3991(99)00086-5.

70. Sinsky, Christine, Lacey Colligan, Ling Li, Mirela Prgomet, Sam Reynolds, Lindsey Goeders, Johanna Westbrook, Michael Tutty, and George Blike. 2016. "Allocation of Physician Time in Ambulatory Practice: A Time and Motion Study in 4 Specialties." *Annals of Internal Medicine* 165, no. 11: 753–60. https://doi.org/10.7326/M16-0961.

71. Tai-Seale, Ming, Thomas G. McGuire, and Weimin Zhang. 2007. "Time Allocation in Primary Care Office Visits." *Health Services Research* 42, no. 5: 1871–94. https://doi.org/10.1111/j.1475-6773.2006.00689.x.

72. Groves, Michele, Peter O'Rourke, and Heather Alexander. 2003. "The Clinical Reasoning Characteristics of Diagnostic Experts." *Medical Teacher* 25, no. 3: 308–13. https://doi.org/10.1080/01421590310001100427.

73. Beckman, H. B., and R. M. Frankel. 1984. "The Effect of Physician Behavior on the Collection of Data." *Annals of Internal Medicine* 101, no. 5: 692–6. https://doi.org/10.7326/0003-4819-101-5-692.

74. Beckman HB, Frankel RM. 1984. "The Effect of Physician Behavior on the Collection of Data." *Annals of Internal Medicine* 101, no. 5: 692–6. https://doi.org/10.7326/0003-4819-101-5-692.

75. Marvel, M. K., R. M. Epstein, K. Flowers, and H. B. Beckman. 1999. "Soliciting the Patient's Agenda: Have We Improved?." *JAMA* 281, no. 3: 283–7. https://doi.org/10.1001/jama.281.3.283.

76. Tai-Seale, M., McGuire, T. G., & Zhang, W. 2007. "Time Allocation in Primary Care Office Visits." *Health Services Research* 42, no. 5: 1871–94. https://doi.org/10.1111/j.1475-6773.2006.00689.x.

77. Charon, R. 2001, Oct. 17. "The Patient-Physician Relationship. Narrative Medicine: A Model for Empathy, Reflection, Profession, and Trust." *JAMA* 286, no. 15: 1897–902. https://doi.org/10.1001/jama.286.15.1897.

78. *The Dartmouth Atlas of Health Care.* 2010.

79. Zhang, Baohui, Alexi A. Wright, Haiden A. Huskamp, Matthew E. Nilsson, Matthew L. Maciejewski, Craig C. Earle, Susan D. Block, Paul K. Maciejewski, and Holly G. Prigerson. 2009. "Health Care Costs in the Last Week of Life: Associations with End-of-Life Conversations." *Archives of Internal Medicine* 169, no. 5: 480–8. https://doi.org/10.1001/archinternmed.2008.587.

80. Teno, Joan M., Elliott S. Fisher, Mary Beth Hamel, Kristen Coppola, and Neal V. Dawson. 2002. "Medical Care Inconsistent with Patients' Treatment Goals: Association with 1-Year Medicare Resource Use and Survival." *Journal of the American Geriatrics Society* 50, no. 3: 496–500. https://doi.org/10.1046/j.1532-5415.2002.50116.x.

81. Schneiderman, L. J., R. M. Kaplan, E. Rosenberg, and H. Teetzel. 1997. "Do Physicians' Own Preferences for Life-Sustaining Treatment Influence Their Perceptions of Patients' Preferences? A Second Look." *Cambridge Quarterly of Healthcare Ethics: CQ: The International Journal of Healthcare Ethics Committees* 6, no. 2: 131–7. https://doi.org/10.1017/s0963180100007751.

82. Gallo, Joseph J., Joseph B. Straton, Michael J. Klag, Lucy A. Meoni, Daniel P. Sulmasy, Nae-Yuh Wang, and Daniel E. Ford. 2003. "Life-Sustaining Treatments: What Do Physicians Want and Do They Express Their Wishes to Others?." *Journal of the American Geriatrics Society* 51, no. 7: 961–9. https://doi.org/10.1046/j.1365-2389.2003.51309.x.

83. Hofmann, J. C., N. S. Wenger, R. B. Davis, J. Teno, A. F. Connors, N. Desbiens, J. Lynn, and R. S. Phillips. 1997. "Patient Preferences for Communication with Physicians About End-of-Life Decisions. SUPPORT Investigators. Study to Understand Prognoses and Preference

for Outcomes and Risks of Treatment." *Annals of Internal Medicine* 127, no. 1: 1–12. https://doi.org/10.7326/0003-4819-127-1-199707010-00001.

84. Murray, Ken. 2013. "Getting Comfortable with Death and near-Death Experiences: How Doctors Die: A Model for Everyone?." *Missouri Medicine* 110, no. 5: 372–4.

85. Kaplan, A. 2012. "Doctors Die Differently: Why—And How." *Psychiatric Times* 29, no. 6: 1-.

86. Gallo, J. J., Straton, J. B., Klag, M. J., Meoni, L. A., Sulmasy, D. P., Wang, N., & Ford, D. E. 2003. "Life-Sustaining Treatments: What Do Physicians Want and Do They Express Their Wishes to Others?." *Journal of the American Geriatrics Society* 51, no. 7: 961–9. https://doi.org/10.1046/j.1365-2389.2003.51309.x.

87. Lown, Beth A., William D. Clark, and Janice L. Hanson. 2009. "Mutual Influence in Shared Decision Making: A Collaborative Study of Patients and Physicians." *Health Expectations* 12, no. 2: 160–74. https://doi.org/10.1111/j.1369-7625.2008.00525.x.

CHAPTER 10. CONFESSIONS

88. "Vitamin B12 – Health Professional Fact Sheet", Accessed September 18, 2022. https://ods.od.nih.gov/factsheets/VitaminB12-HealthProfessional/#en1.

89. Reynolds, Edward. 2006. "Vitamin B12, Folic Acid, and the Nervous System." *Lancet. Neurology* 5, no. 11: 949–60. https://doi.org/10.1016/S1474-4422(06)70598-1.

90. Levy, Andrea Gurmankin, Aaron M. Scherer, Brian J. Zikmund-Fisher, Knoll Larkin, Geoffrey D. Barnes, and Angela Fagerlin. 2018. "Prevalence of and Factors Associated with Patient Nondisclosure of Medically Relevant Information to Clinicians." *JAMA Network Open* 1, no. 7: e185293. https://doi.org/10.1001/jamanetworkopen.2018.5293.

91. Curry Le Richardson, A., H. Xiao et al. 2013. "Nondisclosure of Smoking Status to Health Care Providers Among Current and Former Smokers in the United States." *Health Education & Behavior* 40: 206–15.

92. Levy, A. G., Scherer, A. M., Zikmund-Fisher, B. J., Larkin, K., Barnes, G. D., & Fagerlin, A. Prevalence of and Factors Associated with Patient Nondisclosure of Medically Relevant Information to Clinicians. *JAMA Network Open*, 2018;*1*(7), e185293–e185293.

93. Agaku, Israel T, Akinyele O Adisa, Olalekan A Ayo-Yusuf, and Gregory N Connolly. 2014. "Concern about Security and Privacy, and Perceived Control over Collection and Use of Health Information Are Related to Withholding of Health Information from Healthcare Providers." *Journal of the American Medical Informatics Association* 21 (2): 374–78. https://doi.org/10.1136/amiajnl-2013-002079.

94. "Health Effects of Cigarette Smoking." *CDC*, Accessed November 6, 2022. https://www.cdc.gov/tobacco/data_statistics/fact_sheets/health_effects/effects_cig_smoking/index.htm.

95. "Deaths from Excessive Alcohol Use in the United States." *CDC*, Accessed September 18, 2022. https://www.cdc.gov/alcohol/features/excessive-alcohol-deaths.html.

96. Friedmann, P. D., D. McCullough, M. H. Chin, and R. Saitz. 2000 Feb. "Screening and Intervention for Alcohol Problems. A National Survey of Primary Care Physicians and Psychiatrists." *Journal of General Internal Medicine* 15, no. 2: 84–91. https://doi.org/10.1046/j.1525-1497.2000.03379.x.

97. Hasin, Deborah S., and Bridget F. Grant. 2015. "The National Epidemiologic Survey on Alcohol and Related Conditions (NESARC) Waves 1 and 2: Review and Summary of Findings."

Social Psychiatry & Psychiatric Epidemiology 50, no. 11: 1609–40. https://doi.org/10.1007/s00127-015-1088-0.

98. Boehnke, Kevin F., Evangelos Litinas, Brianna Worthing, Lisa Conine, and Daniel J. Kruger. 2021. "Communication Between Healthcare Providers and Medical Cannabis Patients Regarding Referral and Medication Substitution." *Journal of Cannabis Research* 3, no. 1, 1–9: 2. https://doi.org/10.1186/s42238-021-00058-0.

99. Azcarate, Patrick M., Alysandra J. Zhang, Salomeh Keyhani, Stacey Steigerwald, Julie H. Ishida, and Beth E. Cohen. 2020. "Medical Reasons for Marijuana Use, Forms of Use, and Patient Perception of Physician Attitudes Among the US Population." *Journal of General Internal Medicine* 35, no. 7: 1979–86. https://doi.org/10.1007/s11606-020-05800-7.

100. Filbey, Francesca M., Sina Aslan, Vince D. Calhoun, Jeffrey S. Spence, Eswar Damaraju, Arvind Caprihan, and Judith Segall. 2014. "Long-Term Effects of Marijuana Use on the Brain." In *Proceedings of the National Academy of Sciences of the United States of America.* Dallas: Center for BrainHealth, University of Texas, TX 75235. Albuquerque: Mind Research Network, NM 87106 111, no. 47: 16913–8. https://doi.org/10.1073/pnas.1415297111.

101. Levy, Andrea Gurmankin, Aaron M. Scherer, Brian J. Zikmund-Fisher, Knoll Larkin, Geoffrey D. Barnes, and Angela Fagerlin. 2018. "Prevalence of and Factors Associated with Patient Nondisclosure of Medically Relevant Information to Clinicians." *JAMA Network Open* 1, no. 7: e185293. https://doi.org/10.1001/jamanetworkopen.2018.5293.

102. Saxe, Gordon A., Lisa Madlensky, Sheila Kealey, David P H P. H. Wu, Karen L. Freeman, and John P. Pierce. 2008. "Disclosure to Physicians of CAM Use by Breast Cancer Patients: Findings from the Women's Healthy Eating and Living Study." *Integrative Cancer Therapies* 7, no. 3: 122–9. https://doi.org/10.1177/1534735408323081.

103. Levy, Andrea Gurmankin, Aaron M. Scherer, Brian J. Zikmund-Fisher, Knoll Larkin, Geoffrey D. Barnes, and Angela Fagerlin. 2018. "Prevalence of and Factors Associated with Patient Nondisclosure of Medically Relevant Information to Clinicians." *JAMA Network Open* 1, no. 7: e185293. https://doi.org/10.1001/jamanetworkopen.2018.5293.

CHAPTER 11. CALL OUT THE RED FLAGS

104. Hampton, J. R., M. J. G. Harrison, J. R. A. Mitchell, J. S. Prichard, and C. Seymour. 1975. "Relative Contributions of History-Taking, Physical Examination and Laboratory Investigation to Diagnosis and Management of Medical Outpatients." *BMJ* 2, no. 5969: 486–9. https://doi.org/10.1136/bmj.2.5969.486.

105. Shogilev, Daniel J., Nicolaj Duus, Stephen R. Odom, and Nathan I. Shapiro. 2014. "Diagnosing Appendicitis: Evidence-Based Review of the Diagnostic Approach in 2014." *Western Journal of Emergency Medicine* 15, no. 7: 859–71. https://doi.org/10.5811/westjem.2014.9.21568.

106. Humes, D. J., and J. Simpson. 2006, Sept. 9. "Acute Appendicitis." *BMJ* 333, no. 7567: 530–4. https://doi.org/10.1136/bmj.38940.664363.AE.

107. Ramanayake, R. P. J. C., and B. M. T. K. Basnayake. 2018. "Evaluation of Red Flags Minimizes Missing Serious Diseases in Primary Care." *Journal of Family Medicine & Primary Care* 7, no. 2: 315–8. https://doi.org/10.4103/jfmpc.jfmpc_510_15.

108. Costa, P. T., and R. R. McCrae. 1985. "Hypochondriasis, Neuroticism, and Aging: When Are Somatic Complaints Unfounded?." *American Psychologist* 40, no. 1: 19–28. https://doi.org/10.1037//0003-066x.40.1.19.

109. Ristvedt, Stephen L., and Kathryn M. Trinkaus. 2005. "Psychological Factors Related to Delay in Consultation for Cancer Symptoms." *Psycho-Oncology* 14, no. 5: 339–50. https://doi.org/10.1002/pon.850.

110. Taber, Jennifer M., Bryan Leyva, and Alexander Persoskie. 2015. "Why Do People Avoid Medical Care? A Qualitative Study Using National Data." *Journal of General Internal Medicine* 30, no. 3: 290–7. https://doi.org/10.1007/s11606-014-3089-1.

111. Taber, Jennifer M., Bryan Leyva, and Alexander Persoskie. "Why Do People Avoid Medical Care? A Qualitative Study Using National Data", 290.

CHAPTER 12. THE DIAGNOSTIC JOURNEY

112. Ladizinski, Barry, and Daniel G. Federman. 2013. "Trousseau Syndrome." *CMAJ: Canadian Medical Association Journal* 185, no. 12: 1063. https://doi.org/10.1503/cmaj.121344.

113. Luck. "Definition of Luck by Merriam-Webster", Accessed April 28, 2021. https://www.merriam-webster.com/dictionary/luck.

114. Nagel, T. 2012. *Mortal Questions. Vol Canto Edition.* Accessed April 28, 2021. Cambridge University Press.

115. Fredriksen, Stale. 2005, Oct. "Luck, Risk, and Blame." *Journal of Medicine & Philosophy* 30, no. 5: 535–53. https://doi.org/10.1080/03605310500253105.

116. Hampton, J. R., M. J. G. Harrison, J. R. A. Mitchell, J. S. Prichard, and C. Seymour. 1975. "Relative Contributions of History-Taking, Physical Examination and Laboratory Investigation to Diagnosis and Management of Medical Outpatients." *BMJ* 2, no. 5969: 486–9. https://doi.org/10.1136/bmj.2.5969.486.

117. Reilly, Brendan M. 2003. "Physical Examination in the Care of Medical Inpatients: An Observational Study." *Lancet* 362, no. 9390: 1100–5. https://doi.org/10.1016/S0140-6736(03)14464-9.

118. "Committee on Diagnostic Error in Health Care; Board on Health Care Services; Institute of Medicine; The National Academies of Sciences, Engineering, and Medicine; Balogh EP, Miller BT, Ball JR." *Improving Diagnosis in Health Care.* Washington, (DC): National Academies Press. 2015 Dec. 29.

119. How doctors choose which specialists they refer to. Accessed September 26, 2022. https://www.kevinmd.com/2010/05/doctors-choose-specialists-refer.html

120. "The Hidden System That Explains How Your Doctor Makes Referrals." WSJ. Accessed September 26, 2022. https://www.wsj.com/articles/the-hidden-system-that-explains-how-your-doctor-makes-referrals-11545926166

121. "The Hidden System That Explains How Your Doctor Makes Referrals."

122. Marewski, Julian N., and Gerd Gigerenzer. 2012. "Heuristic Decision Making in Medicine." *Dialogues in Clinical Neuroscience* 14, no. 1: 77–89. https://doi.org/10.31887/DCNS.2012.14.1/jmarewski.

123. Elstein, A. S. 1999. "Heuristics and Biases: Selected Errors in Clinical Reasoning." *Academic Medicine* 74, no. 7: 791–4. https://doi.org/10.1097/00001888-199907000-00012.

CHAPTER 13. YOUR BODY TELLS THE STORY

124. "MedlinePlus Medical Encyclopedia." Accessed December 24, 2021. https://medlineplus.gov/ency/article/002226.htm

125. Kumar, Bharat, Kristi Ferguson, Melissa Swee, and Manish Suneja. 2021. "Diagnostic

Reasoning by Expert Clinicians: What Distinguishes Them from Their Peers?." *Cureus* 13, no. 11: e19722. https://doi.org/10.7759/cureus.19722.

126. Jauhar, Sandeep. 2006. "The Demise of the Physical Exam." *New England Journal of Medicine* 354, no. 6: 548–51. https://doi.org/10.1056/NEJMp068013.

127. Reilly, Brendan M. 2003. "Physical Examination in the Care of Medical Inpatients: An Observational Study." *Lancet* 362, no. 9390: 1100–5. https://doi.org/10.1016/S0140-6736(03)14464-9.

128. Anderson, Joel G., and Ann Gill Taylor. 2011. "Effects of Healing Touch in Clinical Practice: A Systematic Review of Randomized Clinical Trials." *Journal of Holistic Nursing* 29, no. 3: 221–8. https://doi.org/10.1177/0898010110393353.

129. Bloomfield, H. E., and T. J. Wilt. 2011 Oct. "Evidence Brief: Role of the Annual Comprehensive Physical Examination in the Asymptomatic Adult" [Internet]. Washington, (DC): Department of Veterans Affairs. US.

130. Vital Signs (Body Temperature, Pulse Rate, Respiration Rate, Blood Pressure) | Johns Hopkins Medicine, Accessed November 14, 2022. https://www.hopkins-medicine.org/health/conditions-and-diseases/vital-signs-body-temperature-pulse-rate-respiration-rate-blood-pressure.

131. "Adult BMI Calculator | Healthy Weight, Nutrition, and Physical Activity." *CDC*, Accessed November 14, 2022. https://www.cdc.gov/healthyweight/assessing/bmi/adult_bmi/english_bmi_calculator/bmi_calculator.html.

132. "Assessing Your Weight | Healthy Weight, Nutrition, and Physical Activity." *CDC*, Accessed November 14, 2022. https://www.cdc.gov/healthyweight/assessing/index.html.

133. *Skin Cancer Screening* (PDQ®), patient version, Accessed October 1, 2022. https://www.cancer.gov/types/skin/patient/skin-screening-pdq. NCI.

134. Roth, Mara Y., Joann G. Elmore, Joyce P. Yi-Frazier, Lisa M. Reisch, Natalia V. Oster, and Diana L. Miglioretti. 2011. "Self-Detection Remains a Key Method of Breast Cancer Detection for U.S. Women." *Journal of Women's Health* 20, no. 8: 1135–9, Accessed 12/21/2021. https://www.cancer.org/cancer/breast-cancer/screening-tests-and-early-detection/american-cancer-society-recommendations-for-the-early-detection-of-breast-cancer.html. https://doi.org/10.1089/jwh.2010.2493.

135. Accessed December 21, 2021 https://www.cancer.org/cancer/breast-cancer/screening-tests-and-early-detection/american-cancer-society-recommendations-for-the-early-detection-of-breast-cancer.html

136. "Breast Self-Exam: How to Perform, What to Look For," Accessed November 14, 2022. https://my.clevelandclinic.org/health/diagnostics/3990-breast-self-exam

137. Aberger, Michael, Bradley Wilson, Jeffrey M. Holzbeierlein, Tomas L. Griebling, and Ajay K. Nangia. 2014. "Testicular Self-Examination and Testicular Cancer: A Cost-Utility Analysis." *Cancer Medicine* 3, no. 6: 1629–34. https://doi.org/10.1002/cam4.318.

138. "Testicular Exam", Accessed November 14, 2022. https://www.mayoclinic.org/tests-procedures/testicular-exam/about/pac-20385252. Mayo Clinic Publications.

139. Scannapieco, Frank A., and Albert Cantos. 2016 Oct. "Oral Inflammation and Infection, and Chronic Medical Diseases: Implications for the Elderly." *Periodontology 2000* 72, no. 1: 153–75. https://doi.org/10.1111/prd.12129.

140. Iwasaki, Masanori, Wenche S. Borgnakke, Akihiro Yoshihara, Kayoko Ito, Hiroshi Ogawa, Kaname Nohno, Misuzu Sato, Kumiko Minagawa, Toshihiro Ansai, and Hideo Miyazaki.

2018 Jun. "Hyposalivation and 10-Year All-Cause Mortality in an Elderly Japanese Population." *Gerodontology* 35, no. 2: 87–94. https://doi.org/10.1111/ger.12319.

141. Dörfer, Christof, Christoph Benz, Jun Aida, and Guillaume Campard. 2017. "The Relationship of Oral Health with General Health and NCDs: A Brief Review." *International Dental Journal* 67, no. Suppl 2 Suppl. 2: 14–8. https://doi.org/10.1111/idj.12360.

CHAPTER 14. NOT ALL TESTS ARE NECESSARY

142. Maxim, L. Daniel, Ron Niebo, and Mark J. Utell. 2014. "Screening Tests: A Review with Examples." *Inhalation Toxicology* 26, no. 13: 811–28. https://doi.org/10.3109/08958378.201 4.955932.

143. Freedman, Danielle B. 2015. "Towards Better Test Utilization – Strategies to Improve Physician Ordering and Their Impact on Patient Outcomes." *EJIFCC* 26, no. 1: 15–30.

144. Young, P. L., and L. Olsen. 2010. *The Healthcare Imperative: Lowering Costs and Improving Outcomes: Workshop Series Summary*. Washington, DC: The National Academies Press.

145. Mello, Michelle M., Amitabh Chandra, Atul A. Gawande, and David M. Studdert. 2010. "National Costs of the Medical Liability System.". *Health Affairs* 29, no. 9: 1569–77. https:// doi.org/10.1377/hlthaff.2009.0807.

146. "Choosing Wisely.", Accessed November 14, 2022. https://www.choosingwisely.org/ patient-resources/

147. Shrank, W. H., T. L. Rogstad, and N. Parekh. *Waste in the US Health Care System: Estimated Costs and Potential for Savings. JAMA. Published Online October 7, 2019.*

148. *Recommendation: Cervical Cancer: Screening*, Accessed October 1, 2022. https://www.uspreventiveservicestaskforce.org/uspstf/recommendation/cervical-cancer-screening. United States Preventive Services Task Force.

149. Rank, Brian. 2008. "Executive Physicals — Bad Medicine on Three Counts." *New England Journal of Medicine* 359, no. 14: 1424–5. https://doi.org/10.1056/NEJMp0806270.

150. *Recommendation: Cardiovascular Disease Risk: Screening with Electrocardiography*, Accessed May 16, 2021. https://www.uspreventiveservicestaskforce.org/uspstf/recommendation/cardiovascular-disease-risk-screening-with-electrocardiography. United States Preventive Services Task Force.

151. Guirguis-Blake, Janelle M., Corinne V. Evans, Nadia Redmond, and Jennifer S. Lin. 2018. "Screening for Peripheral Artery Disease Using the Ankle-Brachial Index Updated Evidence Report and Systematic Review for the US Preventive Services Task Force." *JAMA* 320, no. 2: 184–96. https://doi.org/10.1001/jama.2018.4250.

152. Korenstein, Deborah, Maha Mamoor, and Peter B. Bach. 2019. "Preventive Services Offered in Executive Physicals at Top-Ranked Hospitals." *JAMA* 322, no. 11: 1101–3. https://doi. org/10.1001/jama.2019.10563.

153. Beutler, Ernest, and Carol West. 2005. "Hematologic Differences Between African-Americans and Whites: The Roles of Iron Deficiency and α-Thalassemia on Hemoglobin Levels and Mean Corpuscular Volume." *Blood* 106, no. 2: 740–5. https://doi.org/10.1182/blood-2005-02-0713.

154. Nam, Hae-Sung, Sun-Seog Kweon, Jin-Su Choi, Joseph M. Zmuda, P. C. Leung, Li-Yung Lui, Deanna D. Hill, Alan L. Patrick, and Jane A. Cauley. 2013. "Racial/Ethnic Differences in Bone Mineral Density Among Older Women." *Journal of Bone & Mineral Metabolism* 31, no. 2: 190–8. https://doi.org/10.1007/s00774-012-0402-0.

155. Wians, F. H. 2009. "Clinical Laboratory Tests: Which, Why, and What Do the Results Mean?." *Laboratory Medicine* 40, no. 2: 105–13. https://doi.org/10.1309/LM404L0HHUTWWUDD.

156. "Screening Tests for Ovarian Cancer." *Choosing Wisely*, Accessed January 14, 2023. https://www.choosingwisely.org/patient-resources/screening-tests-for-ovarian-cancer/

157. Moss, E. L., J. Hollingworth, and T. M. Reynolds. 2005. "The Role of CA125 in Clinical Practice." *Journal of Clinical Pathology* 58, no. 3: 308–12. https://doi.org/10.1136/jcp.2004.018077.

CHAPTER 15. TOO MUCH MEDICINE, TOO LITTLE CARE

158. Rogers, Wendy A. 2014. "Avoiding the Trap of Overtreatment." *Medical Education* 48, no. 1: 12–4. https://doi.org/10.1111/medu.12371.

159. Ooi, Kanny. 2020. "The Pitfalls of Overtreatment: Why More Care Is Not Necessarily Beneficial." *Asian Bioethics Review* 12, no. 4: 399–417. https://doi.org/10.1007/s41649-020-00145-z.

160. Berwick, Donald M., and Andrew D. Hackbarth. 2012. "Eliminating Waste in U.S. Health Care." *JAMA* 307, no. 14: 1513–6. https://doi.org/10.1001/jama.2012.362.

161. Chen, Candice, Stephen Petterson, Robert Phillips, Andrew Bazemore, and Fitzhugh Mullan. 2014. "Spending Patterns in Region of Residency Training and Subsequent Expenditures for Care Provided by Practicing Physicians for Medicare Beneficiaries." *JAMA* 312, no. 22: 2385–93. https://doi.org/10.1001/jama.2014.15973.

162. Kearney, Matt, Julian Treadwell, and Martin Marshall. 2017. "Overtreatment and Undertreatment: Time to Challenge Our Thinking." *British Journal of General Practice* 67, no. 663: 442–3. https://doi.org/10.3399/bjgp17X692657.

163. Cardona-Morrell, M., Jch Kim, R. M. Turner, M. Anstey, I. A. Mitchell, and K. Hillman. 2016. "Non-beneficial Treatments in Hospital at the End of Life: A Systematic Review on Extent of the Problem." *International Journal for Quality in Health Care* 28, no. 4: 456–69. https://doi.org/10.1093/intqhc/mzw060.

164. Lyu, Heather, Tim Xu, Daniel Brotman, Brandan Mayer-Blackwell, Michol Cooper, Michael Daniel, Elizabeth C. Wick, Vikas Saini, Shannon Brownlee, and Martin A. Makary. 2017. "Overtreatment in the United States." *PLOS ONE* 12, no. 9: e0181970. https://doi.org/10.1371/journal.pone.0181970.

165. Lyu, Heather, Tim Xu, Daniel Brotman, Brandan Mayer-Blackwell, Michol Cooper, Michael Daniel, Elizabeth C. Wick, Vikas Saini, Shannon Brownlee, and Martin A. Makary. "Overtreatment in the United States."

166. "What Is Ozempic and Why Is It Getting so Much Attention? – The New York." *Times*, Accessed December 5, 2022. https://www.nytimes.com/2022/11/22/well/ozempic-diabetes-weight-loss.html.

167. Rao, Dinesh, Gaelyn Scuderi, Chris Scuderi, Reetu Grewal, and Sukhwinder Js Sandhu. 2018. "The Use of Imaging in Management of Patients with Low Back Pain." *Journal of Clinical Imaging Science* 8: 30. https://doi.org/10.4103/jcis.JCIS_16_18.

168. Sasiadek, Marek J., and Joanna Bladowska. 2012. "Imaging of Degenerative Spine Disease – The State of the Art." *Advances in Clinical & Experimental Medicine* 21, no. 2: 133–42.

169. *Choosing Wisely*, Accessed December 5, 2022. https://www.choosingwisely.org/

CHAPTER 16. A PILL FOR EVERYTHING

170. "Prescription Drugs | Health Policy Institute", Accessed October 8, 2022. https://hpi.george-town.edu/rxdrugs/. Georgetown University.

171. "America's Love Affair with Prescription Medication – Consumer Reports", Accessed February 7, 2020. https://www.consumerreports.org/prescription-drugs/too-many-meds-americas-love-affair-with-prescription-medication/#nation

172. "Why EHR Data Interoperability Is Such a Mess in 3 Charts." *Health-care It News*, Accessed March 3, 2022. https://www.healthcareitnews.com/news/why-ehr-data-interoperability-such-mess-3-charts.

173. "Gaps in Individuals' Information Exchange." *Health*, Accessed March 3, 2022. IT.gov. https://www.healthit.gov/data/quickstats/gaps-individuals-information-exchange.

174. "AGS Clinical Practice Guidelines and Recommendations – Geriatrics Care Online", Accessed October 8, 2022. https://geriatricscareonline.org/ProductTypeStore/guidelines-recommendations-position-statements-/8/.

175. *Attitudes and Beliefs About the Use of Over-the-Counter Medicines: A Dose of Reality A National Survey of Consumers and Health Professionals. 2002. http://www.harrisinteractive.com.*

176. Qato, Dima M., Jocelyn Wilder, L. Philip Schumm, Victoria Gillet, and G. Caleb Alexander. 2016, Apr. 1. "Changes in Prescription and Over-The-Counter Medication and Dietary Supplement Use Among Older Adults in the United States, 2005 vs 2011." *JAMA Internal Medicine* 176, no. 4: 473–82. https://doi.org/10.1001/jamainternmed.2015.8581.

177. [177] Nicholson, Kathryn, Moira Stewart, and Amardeep Thind. 2015. "Examining the Symptom of Fatigue in Primary Care: A Comparative Study Using Electronic Medical Records." *Journal of Innovation in Health Informatics* 22, no. 1: 235–43. https://doi.org/10.14236/jhi.v22i1.91.

178. Bensing, J. M., R. L. Hulsman, and K. M. G. Schreurs. 1999. "Gender Differences in Fatigue: Biopsychosocial Factors Relating to Fatigue in Men and Women." *Medical Care* 37, no. 10: 1078–83. https://doi.org/10.1097/00005650-199910000-00011.

179. "Drowsy Driving: Asleep At the Wheel | Features." *CDC*, Accessed February 12, 2020. https://www.cdc.gov/features/dsdrowsydriving/index.html.

180. "Attitudes and Beliefs about the Use of Over-The-Counter Medicines: A Dose of Reality Prepared For: National Council on Patient Information and Education (NCPIE) a National Survey of Consumers and Health Professionals." 2002. https://www.bemedwise.org/wp-content/uploads/2019/12/final_survey.pdf.

181. Zhaang, Ya-Ping, Xiao-Cong Zuo, Zhi-Jun Huang, Ze-Min Kuang, Ming-Gen Lu, Dayue Darrel Duan, and Hong Yuan. 2013. "The Impact of Blood Pressure on Kidney Function in the Elderly: A Cross-Sectional Study." *Kidney & Blood Pressure Research* 38, no. 2–3: 205–16. https://doi.org/10.1159/000355769.

182. Lehault, W. B., and D. M. Hughes. 2017. "Review of the Long-Term Effects of Proton Pump Inhibitors. Federal Practitioner: For the Health Care Professionals of the VA, DoD, and PHS" 34, no. 2: 19–23. 3.

183. Vaezi, Michael F., Yu-Xiao Yang, and Colin W. Howden. 2017, Jul. 1. "Polypharmacy: Evaluating Risks and Deprescribing", Accessed July 19, 2022. https://www.aafp.org/pubs/afp/

issues/2019/0701/p32.html. *Gastroenterology* 153, no. 1: 35–48. https://doi.org/10.1053/j.
gastro.2017.04.047.

184. "Polypharmacy: Evaluating Risks and Deprescribing", Accessed July 19, 2022. https://www.
aafp.org/pubs/afp/issues/2019/0701/p32.html

CHAPTER 17. THE REALITY OF DIETARY SUPPLEMENTS

185. Kantor, Elizabeth D., Colin D. Rehm, Mengmeng Du, Emily White, and Edward L. Giovan-
nucci. Oct. 11, 2016. "Trends in Dietary Supplement Use Among US Adults from 1999–
2012." *JAMA* 316, no. 14: 1464–74. https://doi.org/10.1001/jama.2016.14403.

186. 2017. "CRN Consumer Survey on Dietary Supplements", Accessed April 11, 2021. https://www.
crnusa.org/resources/2017-crn-consumer-survey-dietary-supplements. Council for Responsible Nutrition.

187. Blendon, R. J., C. M. DesRoches, J. M. Benson, M. Brodie, and D. E. Altman. 2001. "Americans' Views on the Use and Regulation of Dietary Supplements." *Archives of Internal Medicine* 161, no. 6: 805–10. https://doi.org/10.1001/archinte.161.6.805.

188. "Multivitamin/mineral Supplements – Health Professional Fact Sheet", Accessed April 14,
2021. https://ods.od.nih.gov/factsheets/MVMS-HealthProfessional/

189. Kennedy, Jae, Chi-Chuan Wang, and Chung-Hsuen Wu. 2008. "Patient Disclosure About
Herb and Supplement Use Among Adults in the US." *Evidence-Based Complementary &
Alternative Medicine: eCAM* 5, no. 4: 451–6. https://doi.org/10.1093/ecam/nem045.

190. Gardiner, Paula, Ekaterina Sadikova, Amanda C. Filippelli, Laura F. White, and Brian W.
Jack. 2015. "Medical Reconciliation of Dietary Supplements: Don't ask, don't tell.". *Patient
Education & Counseling* 98, no. 4: 512–7. https://doi.org/10.1016/j.pec.2014.12.010.

191. Bailey, Regan L., Jaime J. Gahche, Cindy V. Lentino, Johanna T. Dwyer, Jody S. Engel,
Paul R. Thomas, Joseph M. Betz, Christopher T. Sempos, and Mary Frances Picciano. 2011.
"Dietary Supplement Use in the United States, 2003–2006." *Journal of Nutrition* 141, no. 2:
261–6. https://doi.org/10.3945/jn.110.133025.

192. Winslow, L. C., and D. J. Kroll. 1998. "Herbs as Medicines." *Archives of Internal Medicine*
158, no. 20: 2192–9. https://doi.org/10.1001/archinte.158.20.2192.

193. He, Zhe, Laura A. Barrett, Rubina Rizvi, Xiang Tang, Seyedeh Neelufar Payrovnaziri, and
Rui Zhang. 2020. "Assessing the Use and Perception of Dietary Supplements Among Obese
Patients with National Health and Nutrition Examination Survey." *AMIA Summits on Trans-
lational Science Proceedings* 2020: 231–40. /pmc/articles/PMC7233063.

194. Maljaei, Mohammad Bagher, Seyedeh Parisa Moosavian, Omid Mirmosayyeb, Mohammad
Hossein Rouhani, Iman Namjoo, and Asma Bahreini. 2019. "Effect of Celery Extract on
Thyroid Function; Is Herbal Therapy Safe in Obesity?." *International Journal of Preventive
Medicine* 10, no. 1: 55. https://doi.org/10.4103/ijpvm.IJPVM_209_17.

195. Office of Inspector General. 2001. *Adverse Event Reporting for Dietary Supplements: An Inadequate Safety Valve*. Washington, DC: US Department of Health and Human Services, Office
of Inspector General.

196. Velicer, Christine M., and Cornelia M. Ulrich. 2008 Feb. 1. "Vitamin and Mineral Supplement Use Among US Adults After Cancer Diagnosis: A Systematic Review." *Journal of Clinical Oncology* 26, no. 4: 665–73. https://doi.org/10.1200/JCO.2007.13.5905.

197. Guallar, Eliseo, Saverio Stranges, Cynthia Mulrow, Lawrence J. Appel, and Edgar
R. Miller, 3rd. 2013 Dec. 17. "Enough Is Enough: Stop Wasting Money on Vitamin

and Mineral Supplements." *Annals of Internal Medicine* 159, no. 12: 850–1. https://doi. org/10.7326/0003-4819-159-12-201312170-00011.

198. Fortmann, Stephen P., Brittany U. Burda, Caitlyn A. Senger, Jennifer S. Lin, and Evelyn P. Whitlock. 2013 Dec. 17. "Vitamin and Mineral Supplements in the Primary Prevention of Cardiovascular Disease and Cancer: An Updated Systematic Evidence Review for the U.S. Preventive Services Task Force." *Annals of Internal Medicine* 159, no. 12: 824–34. https://doi. org/10.7326/0003-4819-159-12-201312170-00729.

199. Ziegler, E. E., and L. J. Filer Jr. 1996. *Present Knowledge in Nutrition.* 7th ed., International Life Sciences Institute-Nutrition. 1996. *Foundation.*

200. de Kruijk, J. R., and N. C. Notermans. 2005 Nov. 12. "Sensory Disturbances Caused by Multivitamin Preparations." *Nederlands Tijdschrift voor Geneeskunde* 149, no. 46: 2541–4.

201. Ziegler, E. E., and L. J. Filer Jr. 1996. *Present Knowledge in Nutrition.* 7th ed., International Life Sciences Institute-Nutrition. 1996. *Foundation.*

202. Bairati, Isabelle, François Meyer, Michel Gélinas, André Fortin, Abdenour Nabid, François Brochet, Jean-Philippe Mercier, Bernard Têtu, François Harel, et al. 2005. "Randomized Trial of Antioxidant Vitamins to Prevent Acute Adverse Effects of Radiation Therapy in Head and Neck Cancer Patients." *Journal of Clinical Oncology* 23, no. 24: 5805–13. https:// doi.org/10.1200/JCO.2005.05.514.

203. Miller, Edgar R., 3rd, Roberto Pastor-Barriuso, Darshan Dalal, Rudolph A. Riemersma, Lawrence J. Appel, and Eliseo Guallar. January 4, 2005. "Meta-analysis: High-Dosage Vitamin E Supplementation May Increase All-Cause Mortality." *Annals of Internal Medicine* 142, no. 1: 37–46. https://doi.org/10.7326/0003-4819-142-1-200501040-00110

204. Omenn, G. S., G. E. Goodman, M. D. Thornquist, J. Balmes, M. R. Cullen, A. Glass, J. P. Keogh, F. L. Meyskens, B. Valanis, J. H. Williams, et al. 1996 May 2. "Effects of a Combination of Beta Carotene and Vitamin A on Lung Cancer and Cardiovascular Disease." *New England Journal of Medicine* 334, no. 18: 1150–5. https://doi.org/10.1056/NEJM199605023341802.

205. Melhus, H., K. Michaëlsson, A. Kindmark, R. Bergström, L. Holmberg, H. Mallmin, A. Wolk, and S. Ljunghall. 1998 Nov. 15. "Excessive Dietary Intake of Vitamin A Is Associated with Reduced Bone Mineral Density and Increased Risk for Hip Fracture." *Annals of Internal Medicine* 129, no. 10: 770–8. https://doi.org/10.7326/0003-4819-129-10-199811150-00003.

206. Alpha-Tocopherol, Beta Carotene Cancer Prevention Study Group. "The Effect of Vitamin E and Beta Carotene on the Incidence of Lung Cancer and Other Cancers in Male Smokers." April 15, 1994. *New England Journal of Medicine* 330, no. 15: 1029–35. https://doi. org/10.1056/NEJM199404143301501.

207. Rapola, J. M., J. Virtamo, J. K. Haukka, O. P. Heinonen, D. Albanes, P. R. Taylor, and J. K. Huttunen. 1996 Mar. 6. "Effect of Vitamin E and Beta Carotene on the Incidence of Angina Pectoris. A Randomized, Double-Blind, Controlled Trial." *JAMA* 275, no. 9: 693–8. https:// doi.org/10.1001/jama.1996.03530330037026.

208. Melhus, H., K. Michaëlsson, A. Kindmark, R. Bergström, L. Holmberg, H. Mallmin, A. Wolk, and S. Ljunghall. 1998. "Excessive Dietary Intake of Vitamin A Is Associated with Reduced Bone Mineral Density and Increased Risk for Hip Fracture." *Annals of Internal Medicine* 129, no. 10: 770–8. https://doi.org/10.7326/0003-4819-129-10-199811150-00003.

209. Barton, James C., Pauline L. Lee, Carol West, and Sylvia S. Bottomley. 2006. "Iron Overload and Prolonged Ingestion of Iron Supplements: Clinical Features and Mutation Analysis of Hemochromatosis-Associated Genes in Four Cases." *American Journal of Hematology* 81, no. 10: 760–7. https://doi.org/10.1002/ajh.20714.

210. Swanson, Christine A. 2003. "Iron Intake and Regulation: Implications for Iron Deficiency and Iron Overload." *Alcohol* 30, no. 2: 99–102. https://doi.org/10.1016/s0741-8329(03)00103-4.

211. Mullaicharam, A., and N. St. Halligudi. 2018. "St John's Wort (Hypericum perforatum L.): A Review of Its Chemistry, Pharmacology and Clinical Properties." *International Journal of Research in Phytochemical & Pharmacological Sciences* 1, no. 1: 5–11. https://doi.org/10.33974/ijrpps.v1i1.7.

212. Camire, M. E., and M. A. Kantor. 1999. "Dietary Supplements: Nutritional and Legal Considerations." *Food Technology* 53, no. 7: 87–96.

213. "Using Dietary Supplements Wisely", Accessed March 14, 2022. https://www.nccih.nih.gov/health/using-dietary-supplements-wisely. NCCIH.

214. Brown, Amy Christine. 2017. "An Overview of Herb and Dietary Supplement Efficacy, Safety and Government Regulations in the United States with Suggested Improvements. Part 1 of 5 Series." *Food & Chemical Toxicology* 107, no. A: 449–71. https://doi.org/10.1016/j.fct.2016.11.001.

215. "Current Good Manufacturing Practices (CGMPs) for Food and Dietary Supplements", Accessed December 4, 2022. https://www.fda.gov/food/guidance-regulation-food-and-dietary-supplements/current-good-manufacturing-practices-cgmps-food-and-dietary-supplements. FDA.

216. "Facts About the Current Good Manufacturing Practices (CGMPs)", Accessed December 4, 2022.https://www.fda.gov/drugs/pharmaceutical-quality-resources/facts-about-current-good-manufacturing-practices-cgmps. FDA.

217. "Certified for Sport® FAQs CERTIFIED FOR SPORT® FREQUENTLY ASKED QUESTIONS 1." *What Is the Purpose of the Certified for Sport® Program?* http://www.nsfsport.com.

218. "Dietary Supplements & Herbal Medicines", Accessed December 4, 2022. https://www.usp.org/dietary-supplements-herbal-medicines. USP.

219. "Third-party Certifications for Supplements." *Fullscript*, Accessed December 4, 2022. https://fullscript.com/blog/third-party-certifications

220. Adler, S. R., and J. R. Fosket. 1999. "Disclosing Complementary and Alternative Medicine Use in the Medical Encounter: a Qualitative Study in Women with Breast Cancer." *Journal of Family Practice* 48, no. 6: 453–8.

221. Ashar, Bimal H., Tasha N. Rice, and Stephen D. Sisson. 2007. "Physicians' Understanding of the Regulation of Dietary Supplements." *Archives of Internal Medicine* 167, no. 9: 966–1000. https://doi.org/10.1001/archinte.167.9.966.

222. Ashar, Bimal H., Tasha N. Rice, and Stephen D. Sisson. 2007. "Physicians' Understanding of the Regulation of Dietary Supplements." *Archives of Internal Medicine* 167, no. 9: 966–969. https://doi.org/10.1001/archinte.167.9.966.

223. Corbin Winslow, Lisa, and Howard Shapiro. 2002. "Physicians Want Education About Complementary and Alternative Medicine to Enhance Communication with Their Patients." *Archives of Internal Medicine* 162, no. 10: 1176–81. https://doi.org/10.1001/archinte.162.10.1176.

224. Cellini, Matthew, Selasi Attipoe, Paul Seales, Robert Gray, Andrew Ward, Mark Stephens, and Patricia A. Deuster. 2013. "Dietary Supplements: Physician Knowledge and Adverse Event Reporting." *Medicine & Science in Sports & Exercise* 45, no. 1: 23–8. https://doi.org/10.1249/MSS.0b013e318269904f

225. Kwak, Grace, Kimberly Gardner, Bolanle Bolaji, Sarah Franklin, Maung Aung, and Pauline E. Jolly. 2021. "Knowledge, Attitudes and Practices Among Healthcare Professionals Regarding

Complementary Alternative Medicine Use by Patients with Hypertension and Type 2 Diabetes Mellitus in Western Jamaica." *Complementary Therapies in Medicine* 57: 102666. https://doi.org/10.1016/j.ctim.2021.102666.

226. "What is Integrative Medicine?", Accessed March 13, 2022. https://integrativemedicine.arizona.edu/about/definition.html. Andrew Weil Center for Integrative Medicine

227. Harris, P. E., K. L. Cooper, C. Relton, and K. J. Thomas. 2012. "Prevalence of Complementary and Alternative Medicine (CAM) Use by the General Population: A Systematic Review and Update." *International Journal of Clinical Practice* 66, no. 10: 924–39. https://doi.org/10.1111/j.1742-1241.2012.02945.x.

228. "Dietary Supplement Products and Ingredients", Accessed November 20, 2022. https://www.fda.gov/food/dietary-supplements/dietary-supplement-products-ingredients. FDA.

229. "Dietary Supplement Fact Sheets", Accessed November 20, 2022. https://ods.od.nih.gov/factsheets/list-all/

230. *Independent Tests and Reviews of Vitamin, Mineral, and Herbal Supplements – ConsumerLab.com*, Accessed November 20, 2022. https://www.consumerlab.com/.

CHAPTER 18. TO ERR IS HUMAN

231. Croskerry, Pat. 2009. "A Universal Model of Diagnostic Reasoning." *Academic Medicine* 84, no. 8: 1022–8. https://doi.org/10.1097/ACM.0b013e3181ace703.=

232. Marewski, Julian N., and Gerd Gigerenzer. 2012. "Heuristic Decision Making in Medicine." *Dialogues in Clinical Neuroscience* 14, no. 1: 77–89. https://doi.org/10.31887/DCNS.2012.14.1/jmarewski.

233. Tversky, A., and D. Kahneman. 1974. "Judgment Under Uncertainty: Heuristics and Biases." *Science* 185, no. 4157: 1124–31. https://doi.org/10.1126/science.185.4157.1124.

234. Verma, Amol A., Fahad Razak, and Allan S. Detsky. 2014, Feb. 12. "Understanding Choice: Why Physicians Should Learn Prospect Theory." *JAMA* 311, no. 6: 571–2. https://doi.org/10.1001/jama.2013.285245.

235. Savioni, Lucrezia, and Stefano Triberti. 2020 Oct. 28. "Cognitive Biases in Chronic Illness and Their Impact on Patients' Commitment." *Frontiers in Psychology* 11: 579455. https://doi.org/10.3389/fpsyg.2020.579455.

236. Siegel, Rebecca L., Stacey A. Fedewa, William F. Anderson, Kimberly D. Miller, Jiemin Ma, Philip S. Rosenberg, and Ahmedin Jemal. 2017. "Colorectal Cancer Incidence Patterns in the United States, 1974–2013." *Journal of the National Cancer Institute* 109, no. 8. https://doi.org/10.1093/jnci/djw322.

237. Kohn, L. T., J. M. Corrigan, and M. S. Donaldson, eds. 1999. *To Err Is Human: Building a Safer Health System*. Washington, DC: National Academy Press, Institute of Medicine.

238. Croskerry, Pat. 2010. "To Err Is Human — and Let's Not Forget It." *CMAJ: Canadian Medical Association Journal* 182, no. 5: 524. https://doi.org/10.1503/cmaj.100270.

239. 240 Mueller, Frederick O. 2009. "Cheerleading Injuries and Safety." *Journal of Athletic Training* 44, no. 6: 565–6. https://doi.org/10.4085/1062-6050-44.6.565.

240. 241 Mello, Michelle M., Amitabh Chandra, Atul A. Gawande, and David M. Studdert. 2010. "National Costs of the Medical Liability System." *Health Affairs* 29, no. 9: 1569–77. https://doi.org/10.1377/hlthaff.2009.0807

241. Carver, N., V. Gupta, and J. E. Hipskind. updated 2022 Jul. 4. "Medical Error." In *StatPearls* [Internet]. Treasure Island, (FL): StatPearls Publishing: 2022.

242. Ferner, Robin E., and Jeffrey K. Aronson. 2006. "Clarification of Terminology in Medication Errors: Definitions and Classification." *Drug Safety* 29, no. 11: 1011–22. https://doi.org/10.2165/00002018-200629110-00001.

243. Wittich, Christopher M., Christopher M. Burkle, and William L. Lanier. 2014. "Medication Errors: An Overview for Clinicians." *Mayo Clinic Proceedings* 89, no. 8: 1116–25. https://doi.org/10.1016/j.mayocp.2014.05.007.

244. Makaryus, Amgad N., and Eli A. Friedman. 2005. "Patients' Understanding of Their Treatment Plans and Diagnosis at Discharge." *Mayo Clinic Proceedings* 80, no. 8: 991–4. https://doi.org/10.4065/80.8.991.

245. Rozich, John D., Ramona J. Howard, Jane M. Justeson, Patrick D. Macken, Mark E. Lindsay, and Roger K. Resar. 2004. "Standardization as a Mechanism to Improve Safety in Health Care." *Joint Commission Journal on Quality & Safety* 30, no. 1: 5–14. https://doi.org/10.1016/s1549-3741(04)30001-8.

246. Gleason, Kristine M., Jennifer M. Groszek, Carol Sullivan, Denise Rooney, Cynthia Barnard, and Gary A. Noskin. 2004. "Reconciliation of Discrepancies in Medication Histories and Admission Orders of Newly Hospitalized Patients." *American Journal of Health-System Pharmacy* 61, no. 16: 1689–95. https://doi.org/10.1093/ajhp/61.16.1689.

247. Leendertse, Anne J., Antoine C. G. Egberts, Lennart J. Stoker, Patricia M L A M. L. A. van den Bemt, and HARM Study Group. 2008. "Frequency of and Risk Factors for Preventable Medication-Related Hospital Admissions in the Netherlands." *Archives of Internal Medicine* 168, no. 17: 1890–6. https://doi.org/10.1001/archinternmed.2008.3.

CHAPTER 19. A "GOOD" DOCTOR

248. Knight, Lynn Valerie, and Karen Mattick. 2006. "'When I first came here, I thought medicine was black and white': Making Sense of Medicals Students' Ways of Knowing." *Social Science & Medicine* 63, no. 4: 1084–96. https://doi.org/10.1016/j.socscimed.2006.01.017.

249. Zayabalaradjane, Z., B. Abhishekh, M. Ponnusamy, N. Nanda, K. Dharanipragada, and S. Kumar. 2018. "Factors Influencing Medical Students in Choosing Medicine as a Career. Online J Health Allied Scs." 17, no. 4: 5.

250. Heikkilä, Teppo J., Harri Hyppölä, Jukka Vänskä, Tiina Aine, Hannu Halila, Santero Kujala, Irma Virjo, Markku Sumanen, and Kari Mattila. 2015. "Factors Important in the Choice of a Medical Career: A Finnish National Study." *BMC Medical Education* 15, no. 1: 169. https://doi.org/10.1186/s12909-015-0451-x.

251. Landon, Bruce E., James D. Reschovsky, Hoangmai H. Pham, and David Blumenthal. 2006. "Leaving Medicine: The Consequences of Physician Dissatisfaction." *Medical Care* 44, no. 3: 234–42. https://doi.org/10.1097/01.mlr.0000199848.17133.9b.

252. Lambert, T. W., F. Smith, and M. J. Goldacre. 2016. "Changes in Factors Influencing Doctors' Career Choices Between One and Five Years After Graduation: Questionnaire Surveys of UK Doctors." *Journal of the Royal Society of Medicine* 109, no. 11: 416–25. https://doi.org/10.1177/0141076816672432.

253. Friedman, Sam, and Daniel Laurison. 2020. *The Class Ceiling: Why It Pays to Be Privileged.* Policy Press.

254. Zayabalaradjane, Z., B. Abhishekh, M. Ponnusamy, N. Nanda, K. Dharanipragada, and S. Kumar. 2018. "Factors Influencing Medical Students in Choosing Medicine as a Career. Online J Health Allied Scs." 17, no. 4: 5.

255. Dyrbye, Liselotte N., Matthew R. Thomas, and Tait D. Shanafelt. 2006. "Systematic Review

of Depression, Anxiety, and Other Indicators of Psychological Distress Among US and Canadian Medical Students." *Academic Medicine* 81, no. 4: 354–73–37316565188. https://doi.org/10.1097/00001888-200604000-00009.

256. Charlson, Mary E., Jwala Karnik, Mitchell Wong, Charles E. McCulloch, and James P. Hollenberg. 2005. "Does Experience Matter? A Comparison of the Practice of Attendings and Residents." *Journal of General Internal Medicine* 20, no. 6: 497–503. https://doi.org/10.1111/j.1525-1497.2005.0085.x.

257. Choudhry, Niteesh K., Robert H. Fletcher, and Stephen B. Soumerai. 2005. "Systematic Review: The Relationship Between Clinical Experience and Quality of Health Care." *Annals of Internal Medicine* 142, no. 4: 260–73. https://doi.org/10.7326/0003-4819-142-4-200502150-00008.

258. Tsugawa, Yusuke, Joseph P. Newhouse, Alan M. Zaslavsky, Daniel M. Blumenthal, and Anupam B. Jena. 2017. "Physician Age and Outcomes in Elderly Patients in Hospital in the US: Observational Study." *BMJ* 357: j1797. https://doi.org/10.1136/bmj.j1797.

259. Plunkett, Beth A., Priya Kohli, and Magdy P. Milad. 2002. "The Importance of Physician Gender in the Selection of an Obstetrician or a Gynecologist." *American Journal of Obstetrics & Gynecology* 186, no. 5: 926–8. https://doi.org/10.1067/mob.2002.123401.

260. "These Medical Specialties Have the Biggest Gender Imbalances", Accessed April 28, 2022. https://www.ama-assn.org/residents-students/specialty-profiles/these-medical-specialties-have-biggest-gender-imbalances. American Medical Association.

261. Kaiser Family Foundation. 2016. *Distribution of Physicians by Gender*. Menlo Park, CA: Kaiser Family Foundation.

262. Kim, Catherine, Laura N. McEwen, Robert B. Gerzoff, David G. Marrero, Carol M. Mangione, Joseph V. Selby, and William H. Herman. 2005. "Is Physician Gender Associated with the Quality of Diabetes Care?." *Diabetes Care* 28, no. 7: 1594–8. https://doi.org/10.2337/diacare.28.7.1594.

263. Baumhäkel, Magnus, Ulrike Müller, and Michael Böhm. 2009. "Influence of Gender of Physicians and Patients on Guideline-Recommended Treatment of Chronic Heart Failure in a Cross-Sectional Study." *European Journal of Heart Failure* 11, no. 3: 299–303. https://doi.org/10.1093/eurjhf/hfn041.

264. Frank, Erica, Yizchak Dresner, Michal Shani, and Shlomo Vinker. 2013. "The Association Between Physicians' and Patients' Preventive Health Practices." *CMAJ* 185, no. 8: 649–53. https://doi.org/10.1503/cmaj.121028.

265. Franks, Peter, and Klea D. Bertakis. 2003. "Physician Gender, Patient Gender, and Primary Care." *Journal of Women's Health* 12, no. 1: 73–80. https://doi.org/10.1089/154099903321154167.

266. Franks, Peter, and Klea D. Bertakis. "Physician Gender, Patient Gender, and Primary Care", 213-218.

267. Roter, Debra L., Judith A. Hall, and Yutaka Aoki. 2002. "Physician Gender Effects in Medical Communication: A Meta-analytic Review." *JAMA* 288, no. 6: 756–64. https://doi.org/10.1001/jama.288.6.756.

268. Ferguson, Eamonn, David James, and Laura Madeley. 2002. "Factors Associated with Success in Medical School: Systematic Review of the Literature." *BMJ* 324, no. 7343: 952–7. https://doi.org/10.1136/bmj.324.7343.952.

269. Roter, Debra L., Judith A. Hall, and Yutaka Aoki. "Physician Gender Effects in Medical Communication: A Meta-analytic Review", 756-764.

270. Tsugawa, Yusuke, Anupam B. Jena, Jose F. Figueroa, E. John Orav, Daniel M. Blumenthal,

and Ashish K. Jha. 2017. "Comparison of Hospital Mortality and Readmission Rates for Medicare Patients Treated by Male vs Female Physicians." *JAMA Internal Medicine* 177, no. 2: 206–13. https://doi.org/10.1001/jamainternmed.2016.7875.

271. "How IMGs Have Changed the Face of American Medicine", Accessed January 14, 2023. https://www.ama-assn.org/education/international-medical-education/how-imgs-have-changed-face-american-medicine. American Medical Association.

272. Frank, Erica, Yizchak Dresner, Michal Shani, and Shlomo Vinker. "The Association Between Physicians' and Patients' Preventive Health Practices", 649-53.

273. Frank, Erica. 2004. "STUDENTJAMA. Physician Health and Patient Care." *JAMA* 291, no. 5: 637–. https://doi.org/10.1001/jama.291.5.637.

274. Frank, E., D. J. Brogan, A. H. Mokdad, E. J. Simoes, H. S. Kahn, and R. S. Greenberg. 1998. "Health-Related Behaviors of Women Physicians vs Other Women in the United States." *Archives of Internal Medicine* 158, no. 4: 342–8. https://doi.org/10.1001/archinte.158.4.342.

275. Frank, E., D. J. Brogan, A. H. Mokdad, E. J. Simoes, H. S. Kahn, and R. S. Greenberg. "Health-Related Behaviors of Women Physicians vs Other Women in the United States", 342-348

276. Parmar, Malvinder S. 2002 Sept. 28. "What's a Good Doctor and How Do You Make One? ABC of Being a Good Doctor." *BMJ* 325, no. 7366: 711; author reply 711. https://doi.org/10.1136/bmj.325.7366.711.

277. Groopman, Jerome E. 2007. *How Doctors Think*. Houghton Mifflin Company.

278. Kalmoe, Molly C., Matthew B. Chapman, Jessica A. Gold, Andrea M. Giedinghagen, and M. Chapman. 2019. "Physician Suicide: A Call to Action." *Missouri Medicine* 116, no. 3: 211–6.

279. Seys, Deborah, Albert W. Wu, Eva Van Gerven, Arthur Vleugels, Martin Euwema, Massimiliano Panella, Susan D. Scott, James Conway, Walter Sermeus, and Kris Vanhaecht. 2013. "Health Care Professionals as Second Victims After Adverse Events: A Systematic Review." *Evaluation & the Health Professions* 36, no. 2: 135–62. https://doi.org/10.1177/0163278712458918.

280. Agnelli, Giancarlo. 2004. "Prevention of Venous Thromboembolism in Surgical Patients." *Circulation* 110, no. 24 Suppl. 1: IV4–12. https://doi.org/10.1161/01.CIR.0000150639.98514.6c.

281. Hu, Yue-Yung, Megan L. Fix, Nathanael D. Hevelone, Stuart R. Lipsitz, Caprice C. Greenberg, Joel S. Weissman, and J. Shapiro. 2012. "Physicians' Needs in Coping with Emotional Stressors: The Case for Peer Support." *Archives of Surgery*. Chicago, IL 147, no. 3: 212–7. https://doi.org/10.1001/archsurg.2011.312.

282. Seys, Deborah, Albert W. Wu, Eva Van Gerven, Arthur Vleugels, Martin Euwema, Massimiliano Panella, Susan D. Scott, James Conway, Walter Sermeus, and Kris Vanhaecht. "Health Care Professionals as Second Victims After Adverse Events: a Systematic Review."

283. Kalmoe, Molly C., Matthew B. Chapman, Jessica A. Gold, Andrea M. Giedinghagen, and M. Chapman. 2019. "Physician Suicide: A Call to Action." *Missouri Medicine* 116, no. 3: 211–6.

284. Reynolds, F. 2006. "How Doctors Cope with Death." *Archives of Disease in Childhood* 91, no. 9: 727. https://doi.org/10.1136/adc.2005.092015.

CHAPTER 20. HOSPITALS ARE "HOMES" FOR DOCTORS, BUT NOT FOR PATIENTS

285. Neuberger, J. 1999 Jun. 26. "Do We Need a New Word for Patients? Lets Do Away with 'Patients'." *BMJ* 318, no. 7200: 1756–7. https://doi.org/10.1136/bmj.318.7200.1756.

286. Nilmini Wickramasinghe, Latif Al-Hakim, Chris Gonzalez, and Joseph Tan. 2014. *Lean Thinking for Healthcare*. New York, Ny Springer.

287. Gale, Arthur H. 2016. "The Hospital as a Factory and the Physician as an Assembly Line Worker." *Missouri Medicine* 113, no. 1: 7–9.

288. Lateef, Fatimah. 2011. "Patient Expectations and the Paradigm Shift of Care in Emergency Medicine." *Journal of Emergencies, Trauma, & Shock* 4, no. 2: 163–7. https://doi.org/10.4103/0974-2700.82199.

289. Braithwaite, Jeffrey, Jessica Herkes, Kristiana Ludlow, Luke Testa, and Gina Lamprell. 2017, Nov. 1. "Association Between Organisational and Workplace Cultures, and Patient Outcomes: Systematic Review." *BMJ Open* 7, no. 11: e017708. https://doi.org/10.1136/bmjopen-2017-017708.

CHAPTER 21. HOME RULES FOR HOSPITALS

290. Brennan, T. A., L. L. Leape, N. M. Laird, L. Hebert, A. R. Localio, A. G. Lawthers, J. P. Newhouse, P. C. Weiler, and H. H. Hiatt. 1991. "Incidence of Adverse Events and Negligence in Hospitalized Patients. Results of the Harvard Medical Practice Study I." *New England Journal of Medicine* 324, no. 6: 370–6. https://doi.org/10.1056/NEJM199102073240604.

291. Makary, Martin A., and Michael Daniel. 2016 May 3. "Medical Error—The Third Leading Cause of Death in the US." *BMJ* 353: i2139. https://doi.org/10.1136/bmj.i2139.

292. Rodwin, Benjamin A., Victor P. Bilan, Naseema B. Merchant, Catherine G. Steffens, Alyssa A. Grimshaw, Lori A. Bastian, and Craig G. Gunderson. 2020, Jul. 1. "Rate of Preventable Mortality in Hospitalized Patients: A Systematic Review and Meta-analysis." *Journal of General Internal Medicine* 35, no. 7: 2099–106. https://doi.org/10.1007/s11606-019-05592-5.

293. Cross, Sarah H., and Haider J. Warraich. 2019. "Changes in the Place of Death in the United States." *New England Journal of Medicine* 381, no. 24: 2369–70. https://doi.org/10.1056/NEJMc1911892.

294. Braithwaite, Jeffrey, Jessica Herkes, Kristiana Ludlow, Luke Testa, and Gina Lamprell. 2017, Nov. 1. "Association Between Organisational and Workplace Cultures, and Patient Outcomes: Systematic Review." *BMJ Open* 7, no. 11: e017708. https://doi.org/10.1136/bmjopen-2017-017708.

295. Weingart, Saul N., Odelya Pagovich, Daniel Z. Sands, Joseph M. Li, Mark D. Aronson, Roger B. Davis, Russell S. Phillips, and David W. Bates. 2006 Apr. "Patient-Reported Service Quality on a Medicine Unit." *International Journal for Quality in Health Care* 18, no. 2: 95–101. https://doi.org/10.1093/intqhc/mzi087.

296. Sternberg, Esther M. 2010. *Healing Spaces: The Science of Place and Well-Being*. Cambridge, Massachusetts.: Belknap Press Of Harvard University Press

297. Daruna, Jorge Hilarion. 2012. *Introduction to Psychoneuroimmunology*. San Diego: Elsevier Academic Press.

298. Travis, Fred, Laurent Valosek, Arthur Konrad, Janice Link, John Salerno, Ray Scheller, and Sanford Nidich. 2018. "Effect of Meditation on Psychological Distress and Brain Functioning: A Randomized Controlled Study." *Brain & Cognition* 125: 100–5. https://doi.org/10.1016/j.bandc.2018.03.011.

299. Andrade, Gabriel. 2019. "The Ethics of Positive Thinking in Healthcare." *Journal of Medical Ethics & History of Medicine* 12: 18. https://doi.org/10.18502/jmehm.v12i18.2148.

300. Kurtz, Paul. 2013. *The Transcendental Temptation: A Critique of Religion and the Paranormal.* Amherst, NY: Prometheus Books.

CHAPTER 22. HOW TO GET THREE DOCTORS FOR THE PRICE OF ONE

301. Figueroa, Jose F., Yusuke Tsugawa, Jie Zheng, E. John Orav, and Ashish K. Jha. 2016. "Association Between the Value-Based Purchasing Pay for Performance Program and Patient Mortality in US Hospitals: Observational Study." *BMJ* 353: i2214. https://doi.org/10.1136/bmj.i2214.

302. Charlson, Mary E., Jwala Karnik, Mitchell Wong, Charles E. McCulloch, and James P. Hollenberg. 2005. "Does Experience Matter? A Comparison of the Practice of Attendings and Residents." *Journal of General Internal Medicine* 20, no. 6: 497–503. https://doi.org/10.1111/j.1525-1497.2005.0085.x.

303. van der Leeuw, Renée M., Kiki M J M H M. J. M. H. Lombarts, Onyebuchi A. Arah, and Maas Jan Heineman. 2012. "A Systematic Review of the Effects of Residency Training on Patient Outcomes." *BMC Medicine* 10, no. 1: 65. https://doi.org/10.1186/1741-7015-10-65.

CHAPTER 23. HOW TO FIND HEALTHCARE THAT FITS

304. Andersen, R., and J. F. Newman. 2005. "Societal and Individual Determinants of Medical Care Utilization in the United States." *Milbank Quarterly* 83, no. 4.

305. "Patients' Perspectives on the State of Healthcare in America", Accessed March 16, 2022. https://www.ajmc.com/view/patients-perspectives-on-the-state-of-healthcare-in-america.

306. "Unnecessary ED Visits from Chronically Ill Patients Cost $8.3Bn", Accessed July 1, 2021. https://www.modernhealthcare.com/article/20190207/TRANSFORMATION03/190209949/unnecessary-ed-visits-from-chronically-ill-patients-cost-8-3-billion.

307. Hunt, R. C., K. L. DeHart, E. J. Allison, and T. W. Whitley. 1996. "Patient and Physician Perception of Need for Emergency Medical Care: A Prospective and Retrospective Analysis." *American Journal of Emergency Medicine* 14, no. 7: 635–9. https://doi.org/10.1016/S0735-6757(96)90077-7.

308. Kraaijvanger, Nicole, Henk Van Leeuwen, Douwe Rijpsma, and Michael Edwards. 2016. "Motives for Self-Referral to the Emergency Department: A Systematic Review of the Literature." *BMC Health Services Research* 16, no. 1: 685. https://doi.org/10.1186/s12913-016-1935-z.

309. Kraaijvanger, Nicole, Henk Van Leeuwen, Douwe Rijpsma, and Michael Edwards. "Motives for Self-Referral to the Emergency Department: A Systematic Review of the Literature."

310. Sachs, C. J., C. K. Yu, P. C. Nauka, and D. L. Schriger. 2017. "Systems Opportunities to Reduce ED Crowding from Nonemergency Referrals" 33, no. 1: 37–42.

CHAPTER 24. NOT ALL PRACTICES ARE CREATED EQUAL

311. "Total Active Doctors in the U.S. by State." 2021, Accessed April 13, 2022. https://www.statista.com/statistics/186269/total-active-physicians-in-the-us/. Statista.

312. Kurtzman, Ellen T., and Burt S. Barnow. 2017. "A Comparison of Nurse Practitioners, Physician Assistants, and Primary Care Physicians' Patterns of Practice and Quality of Care in Health Centers." *Medical Care* 55, no. 6: 615–22. https://doi.org/10.1097/MLR.0000000000000689.

313. *Compare the Education Gaps Between Primary Care Physicians and Nurse Practitioners.* Retrieved from http://www.aafp.org/online/en/home/media/kits/fp-np.html.

314. Mafi, John N., Christina C. Wee, Roger B. Davis, and Bruce E. Landon. 2016. "Comparing

Use of Low-Value Health Care Services Among US Advanced Practice Clinicians and Physicians." *Annals of Internal Medicine* 165, no. 4: 237–44. https://doi.org/10.7326/M15-2152.

315. "Physician Practice Benchmark Survey", Accessed July 5, 2021. https://www.ama-assn.org/about/research/physician-practice-benchmark-survey. American Medical Association.

316. Casalino, Lawrence P., Michael F. Pesko, Andrew M. Ryan, Jayme L. Mendelsohn, Kennon R. Copeland, Patricia Pamela Ramsay, Xuming Sun, Diane R. Rittenhouse, and Stephen M. Shortell. 2014. "Small Primary Care Physician Practices Have Low Rates of Preventable Hospital Admissions." *Health Affairs (Project Hope)* 33, no. 9: 1680–8. https://doi.org/10.1377/hlthaff.2014.0434.

317. "Mapper—Direct Primary Care." *DPC Frontier*, Accessed November 21, 2022. https://mapper.dpcfrontier.com/.

318. "Common Sense Family Doctor: How Much Administration Does Health Care Really Need?", Accessed April 9, 2022 http://commonsensemd.blogspot.com/2022/02/how-much-administration-does-health.html?utm_source=feedburner&utm_medium=email.

319. "Number of Healthcare Administrators Explodes Since 1970", Accessed April 9, 2022. https://www.athenahealth.com/knowledge-hub/practice-management/expert-forum-rise-and-rise-healthcare-administrator.

320. "70% of Physicians Are Now Employed by Hospitals or Corporations", Accessed April 9, 2022. https://www.beckersasc.com/asc-transactions-and-valuation-issues/70-of-physicians-are-now-employed-by-hospitals-or-corporations.html.

CHAPTER 25. HEALTHCARE CHOICES HINGE ON WHO WE ARE

321. "Generational Divides Influence Doctor–Patient Relationships, Patient Engagement, Study Says." *Healthcare Finance News*, Accessed June 16, 2021. https://www.healthcarefinancenews.com/news/generational-divides-influence-doctor-patient-relationships-patient-engagement-study-says.

322. Park, M. Jane, Tina Paul Mulye, Sally H. Adams, Claire D. Brindis, and Charles E. Irwin. 2006. "The Health Status of Young Adults in the United States." *Journal of Adolescent Health* 39, no. 3: 305–17. https://doi.org/10.1016/j.jadohealth.2006.04.017.

323. Mohler-Kuo, Meichun, Hans Wydler, Ueli Zellweger, and Felix Gutzwiller. 2006. "Differences in Health Status and Health Behaviour Among Young Swiss Adults Between 1993 and 2003." *Swiss Medical Weekly* 136, no. 29–30: 464–72. https://doi.org/10.4414/smw.2006.11322.

324. Marshall, Emily G. 2011. "Do Young Adults Have Unmet Healthcare Needs?" *Journal of Adolescent Health* 49, no. 5: 490–7. https://doi.org/10.1016/j.jadohealth.2011.03.005.

325. Tandon, S. Darius, Beth Marshall, Amy J. Templeman, and Freya L. Sonenstein. 2008. "Health Access and Status of Adolescents and Young Adults Using Youth Employment and Training Programs in an Urban Environment." *Journal of Adolescent Health* 43, no. 1: 30–7. https://doi.org/10.1016/j.jadohealth.2007.12.006.

326. Marshall, Emily G. 2011. "Do Young Adults Have Unmet Healthcare Needs?"

327. "Gen Z Is Aging out of Pediatrics—What Does That Mean for Your Growth Strategy?" n.d. www.advisory.com. Accessed July 7, 2021. https://www.advisory.com/blog/2019/08/gen-z-patients.

328. Davey, Antoinette, Anthea Asprey, Mary Carter, and John L. Campbell. 2013. "Trust, Negotiation, and Communication: Young Adults' Experiences of Primary Care Services." *BMC Family Practice* 14(1), 1–10: 202. https://doi.org/10.1186/1471-2296-14-202.

329. Davey, Antoinette, Anthea Asprey, Mary Carter, and John L. Campbell. 2013. "Trust, Negotiation, and Communication: Young Adults' Experiences of Primary Care Services."

330. "Things to Know About Winning Millennial and Boomer New Patients", Accessed July 13, 2021. https://healthcaresuccess.com/blog/hospital-marketing/21-things-know-winning-millennial-boomer-new-patients.html.

331. "Is Social Media Changing the Doctor–Patient Relationship?", Accessed July 7, 2021 https://www.aafp.org/news/practice-professional-issues/20180608commsurveys.html.

332. "5 trends in healthcare inspired by millennials", Accessed July 13, 2021. https://www.beckershospitalreview.com/hospital-management-administration/5-trends-in-healthcare-inspired-by-millennials.html.

333. "The Patient-Provider Relationship Study: The Ripple Effect", Accessed January 14, 2023. https://www.solutionreach.com/rethinking-the-patient-provider-relationship?source_url=https%3A%2F%2Fwww.solutionreach.com%2Frethinking-the-patient-provider-relationship.

334. "Generation X (Gen X) Definition", Accessed July 12, 2021. https://www.investopedia.com/terms/g/generation-x-genx.asp.

335. Zheng, Hui, and Paola Echave. 2021 Nov. 2. "Are Recent Cohorts Getting Worse? Trends in US Adult Physiological Status, Mental Health, and Health Behaviors Across a Century of Birth Cohorts." *American Journal of Epidemiology* 190, no. 11: 2242–55. https://doi.org/10.1093/aje/kwab076.

336. "Survey: Gen X Leads the Charge on Digital Health Adoption." *Business Wire*, Accessed July 12, 2021. https://www.businesswire.com/news/home/20191022005409/en/Survey-Gen-X-Leads-the-Charge-on-Digital-Health-Adoption.

337. Knickman, James R., and Emily K. Snell. 2002. "The 2030 Problem: Caring for Aging Baby Boomers." *Health Services Research* 37, no. 4: 849–84. https://doi.org/10.1034/j.1600-0560.2002.56.x.

CHAPTER 26. CHRONIC ILLNESS AS A PIVOTING POINT

338. Weil, MD, Andrew. 2000. *Spontaneous Healing*. Random House Publishing Group. Kindle Edition.136.

339. Ma, Ying, Qin Xiang, Chaoyang Yan, Hui Liao, and Jing Wang. 2021. "Relationship Between Chronic Diseases and Depression: The Mediating Effect of Pain." *BMC Psychiatry* 21, no. 1: 436. https://doi.org/10.1186/s12888-021-03428-3.

340. Kübler-Ross, E. 1969. *On Death and Dying*. New York: Macmillan Company.

341. Egnew, Thomas R. 2018. "A Narrative Approach to Healing Chronic Illness." *Annals of Family Medicine* 16, no. 2: 160–5. https://doi.org/10.1370/afm.2182.

342. Buss, D. M. 2000. "The Evolution of Happiness." *American Psychologist* 55, no. 1: 15–23. https://doi.org/10.1037/0003-066X.55.1.15.

343. Clear, James. 2018. *Atomic Habits* .Penguin Publishing Group. Kindle Edition.

344. Egnew, Thomas R. "A Narrative Approach to Healing Chronic Illness."

345. Buss, D. M. "The evolution of happiness."

346. "Risk of Stroke Associated with Bypass Surgery Technique Designed to Prevent Organ Damage." 04/22/2010, Accessed August 6, 2022. https://www.hopkinsmedicine.org/news/media/releases/risk_of_stroke_associated_with_bypass_surgery_technique_designed_to_prevent_organ_damage.

347. Gaudino, M., D. J. Angiolillo, A. Di Franco, D. Capodanno, F. Bakaeen, M. E. Farkouh, and D. P. Taggart. 2019. "Stroke After Coronary Artery Bypass Grafting and Percutaneous Coronary Intervention: Incidence, Pathogenesis, and Outcomes." *Journal of the American Heart Association* 8, no. 13: 13032.

348. Tali Sharot. 2012. *The Optimism Bias : A Tour of the Irrationally Positive Brain.* New York: Vintage Books.

349. Dunning, David, Chip Heath, and Jerry M. Suls. "Flawed Self-Assessment: Implications for Health, Education, and the Workplace." 2004. *Psychological Science in the Public Interest* 5, no. 3: 69–106. https://doi.org/10.1111/j.1529-1006.2004.00018.x.

350. Weinstein, N. D. 1980. "Unrealistic Optimism About Future Life Events." *Journal of Personality & Social Psychology* 39, no. 5: 806–20. https://doi.org/10.1037/0022-3514.39.5.806.

351. Larwood, L. 1978. "Swine Flu: A Field Study of Self-Serving Biases." *Journal of Applied Social Psychology* 8, no. 3: 283–9. https://doi.org/10.1111/j.1559-1816.1978.tb00783.x.

352. Seligman, M. E. P., and S. F. Maier. 1967. "Failure to Escape Traumatic Shock." *Journal of Experimental Psychology* 74, no. 1: 1–9. https://doi.org/10.1037/h0024514.

353. "Why Don't Patients Follow Their Doctors' Advice?", Accessed May 14, 2022 https://www.aamc.org/news-insights/why-don-t-patients-follow-their-doctors-advice. AAMC.

354. "15 Badass Sick People Throughout History", Accessed June 4, 2022. https://www.yahoo.com/lifestyle/15-badass-sick-people-throughout-134322690.html.

355. Savioni, Lucrezia, and Stefano Triberti. 2020. "Cognitive Biases in Chronic Illness and Their Impact on Patients' Commitment." *Frontiers in Psychology* 11: 579455. https://doi.org/10.3389/fpsyg.2020.579455.

CHAPTER 27. POWER TO HEAL

356. "Balint Groups – the American Balint Society." n.d. Www.americanbalintsociety.org. Accessed September 28, 2021. https://www.americanbalintsociety.org/content.aspx?page_id=22&club_id=445043&module_id=406070.

357. Kleinman, A. M. 1973. "Some Issues for a Comparative Study of Medical Healing." *International Journal of Social Psychiatry* 19, no. 3: 159–63. https://doi.org/10.1177/002076407301900301.

358. *Webster's New Collegiate Dictionary.* 1976. Springfield, Mass.: G. & C. Merriam Co.

359. McElligott, Deborah. 2010. "Healing: The Journey from Concept to Nursing Practice." *Journal of Holistic Nursing* 28, no. 4: 251–9. https://doi.org/10.1177/0898010110376321.

360. Eisenberg, D. M., R. B. Davis, S. L. Ettner, S. Appel, S. Wilkey, M. Van Rompay, and R. C. Kessler. 1998. "Trends in Alternative Medicine Use in the United States, 1990–1997: Results of a Follow-Up National Survey." *JAMA* 280, no. 18: 1569–75. https://doi.org/10.1001/jama.280.18.1569.

361. Brown, Marie T., and Jennifer K. Bussell. 2011 Apr. "Medication Adherence: WHO Cares?." *Mayo Clinic Proceedings* 86, no. 4: 304–14. https://doi.org/10.4065/mcp.2010.0575.

362. Hsu, Clarissa, William R. Phillips, Karen J. Sherman, Rene Hawkes, and Daniel C. Cherkin. 2008. "Healing in Primary Care: A Vision Shared by Patients, Physicians, Nurses, and Clinical Staff." *Annals of Family Medicine* 6, no. 4: 307–14. https://doi.org/10.1370/afm.838.

363. Lloyd-Jones, Donald M., Yuling Hong, Darwin Labarthe, Dariush Mozaffarian, Lawrence J. Appel, Linda Van Horn, Kurt Greenlund, Stephen Daniels, Graham Nichol, et al., and American Heart Association Strategic Planning Task Force and Statistics Committee. 2010. "Defining and Setting National Goals for Cardiovascular Health Promotion and Disease Reduction:

The American Heart Association's Strategic Impact Goal Through 2020 and Beyond." *Circulation* 121, no. 4: 586–613. https://doi.org/10.1161/CIRCULATIONAHA.109.192703.

364. Eisenberg, D. M., R. B. Davis, S. L. Ettner, S. Appel, S. Wilkey, M. Van Rompay, and R. C. Kessler. "Trends in Alternative Medicine Use in the United States, 1990–1997: Results of a Follow-Up National Survey."

365. "Harvard Food Law Clinic Calls for Greater Nutrition Education in the Medical Field – Harvard Law Today", Accessed May 31, 2022. https://today.law.harvard.edu/harvard-food-law-clinic-calls-for-greater-nutrition-education-in-the-medical-field/.

366. Wolsko, Peter M., David M. Eisenberg, Roger B. Davis, and Russell S. Phillips. 2004. "Use of Mind–Body Medical Therapies: Results of a National Survey." *Journal of General Internal Medicine* 19, no. 1: 43–50. https://doi.org/10.1111/j.1525-1497.2004.21019.x.

367. Salamonsen, Anita. 2013. "Doctor–Patient Communication and Cancer Patients' Choice of Alternative Therapies as Supplement or Alternative to Conventional Care." *Scandinavian Journal of Caring Sciences* 27, no. 1: 70–6. https://doi.org/10.1111/j.1471-6712.2012.01002.x.

368. Kooreman, Peter, and Erik W. Baars. 2012. "Patients Whose GP Knows Complementary Medicine Tend to Have Lower Costs and Live Longer." *European Journal of Health Economics: HEPAC: Health Economics in Prevention & Care* 13, no. 6: 769–76. https://doi.org/10.1007/s10198-011-0330-2.

CHAPTER 28. HEALING BODY AND MIND

369. Video: Dr. Weil's Breathing Exercises: 4-7-8 Breath. Accessed October 17, 2022. https://www.drweil.com/videos-features/videos/breathing-exercises-4-7-8-breath/

370. Russo, Marc A., Danielle M. Santarelli, and Dean O'Rourke. 2017. "The Physiological Effects of Slow Breathing in the Healthy Human." *Breathe* 13, no. 4: 298–309. https://doi.org/10.1183/20734735.009817.

371. Russo, Marc A., Danielle M. Santarelli, and Dean O'Rourke. "The Physiological Effects of Slow Breathing in the Healthy Human", 298.

372. *Tension, Stress and Trauma Release: TRE®*, Accessed May 31, 2022. https://traumaprevention.com/.

373. Berceli, David, Melanie Salmon, Robin Bonifas, and Nkem Ndefo. 2014. "Effects of Self-Induced Unclassified Therapeutic Tremors on Quality of Life Among Non-professional Caregivers: A Pilot Study." *Global Advances in Health & Medicine* 3, no. 5: 45–8. https://doi.org/10.7453/gahmj.2014.032.

374. *Tension, Stress and Trauma Release: TRE®*, Accessed May 31, 2022. https://traumaprevention.com/.

375. Tseui, J. J. 1978. "Eastern and Western Approaches to Medicine." *Western Journal of Medicine* 128, no. 6: 551–7.

376. Aronson, J. 1999. "When I Use a Word." *BMJ* 318, no. 7185: 716. https://doi.org/10.1136/bmj.318.7185.716.

377. Jütte, Robert. 2013. "The Early History of the Placebo." *Complementary Therapies in Medicine* 21, no. 2: 94–7. https://doi.org/10.1016/j.ctim.2012.06.002.

378. Falk, Emily B., Matthew Brook O'Donnell, Christopher N. Cascio, Francis Tinney, Yoona Kang, Matthew D. Lieberman, Shelley E. Taylor, Lawrence An, Kenneth Resnicow, and Victor J. Strecher. 2015. "Self-Affirmation Alters the Brain's Response to Health Messages and

Subsequent Behavior Change." *Proceedings of the National Academy of Sciences of the United States of America* 112, no. 7: 1977–82. https://doi.org/10.1073/pnas.1500247112.

379. Wood, Joanne V., W. Q. Elaine Perunovic, and John W. Lee. 2009. "Positive Self-Statements: Power for Some, Peril for Others.". *Psychological Science* 20, no. 7: 860–6. https://doi.org/10.1111/j.1467-9280.2009.02370.x.

ACKNOWLEDGEMENTS

I owe my gratitude to all doctors and patients whose stories inspired this book, for their undeniable impressions, encouragements and valuable lessons.

I am indebted to the faculty of the University of Arizona Andrew Weil Center of Integrative Medicine for their powerful teaching. Thank you for giving me courage to return to my roots in Eastern Medicine and incorporate it into my clinical practice.

I give thanks for literary inspirations to Drs. Andrew Weil, Victoria Maizes, Jerome Groopman, Abraham Verghese, Danielle Ofri, and Lisa Sanders, whose writings have been models for me. My special gratitude goes to Dr. Clive Brook, whose wisdom and thoughtful approaches to patient-doctor relationship helped the Russian doctor to fit in to American healthcare.

My editors, Claire McGregor and Jess Lomas, were instrumental in patiently editing the manuscript written by the first-time author with English-second language limitations. Rebecca Stahlman graciously brought great insight with her notes and suggestions.

Thank you, Dr. Daniel Cherry, for stepping into a new world of writing with me, for your endless encouragement and support.

My debts are beyond words to my parents, Tatjana Cechanovich and Vladimir Parshin, for their lessons in courage, gratitude and resilience.

ABOUT THE AUTHOR

Maria V Gibson, MD, PhD is a Board-certified family physician, Certified Physician Executive and a Clinical Professor at the University of Arizona, College of Medicine, Phoenix. She grew up in Siberia and received MD and PhD degrees at Siberian State Medical University, where science of Western medicine crossed the ancient wisdom of Eastern medicine from teachers from nearby Far East. Most of her research in Siberia was dedicated to studies of alternative treatments of chronic pelvic pain. Dr. Gibson trained in Family medicine at Duke University and Integrative medicine at the University of Arizona Andrew Weil center of Integrative Medicine.

Her holistic approach and expertise in medical science and integrative lifestyle medicine helped thousands of patients return to health. During her medical, academic, and business career over more than three decades and two continents, Dr. Gibson trained hundreds of medical students, physicians, and medical executives.

She lives in Scottsdale, Arizona with her family and continues practicing and teaching family and integrative medicine.

WWW.DRMARIAGIBSON.COM

www.ingramcontent.com/pod-product-compliance
Lightning Source LLC
Chambersburg PA
CBHW032049020426
42335CB00011B/248